Drug Calculations

Process and Problems for Clinical Practice

Drug Calculations

Process and Problems for Clinical Practice

Meta Brown, R.N., M.Ed.

Director, Division of Nursing,
Gateway Community College,
Phoenix, Arizona;
U.S. Army Reserve

Joyce L. Mulholland, R.N.C., M.A., M.S.

Professor, Division of Nursing,
Gateway Community College,
Phoenix, Arizona

Fourth Edition

illustrated

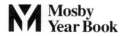
Mosby
Year Book

St. Louis Baltimore Boston Chicago London Philadelphia Sydney Toronto

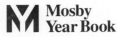

Mosby
Year Book
Dedicated to Publishing Excellence

Senior Editor: Nancy L. Coon
Managing Editor: Susan R. Epstein
Developmental Editor: Suzanne Seeley Wakefield
Project Manager: Gayle May Morris
Book designer: Jeanne Wolfgeher
Cover Photo: Jean Pierre Pieuchot/The Image Bank

As new medical and nursing research and clinical experience broaden our knowledge, changes in treatment and drug therapy are required. The editors and the publisher of this work have made every effort to ensure that the drug dosage schedules herein are accurate and in accord with the standards accepted at the time of publication. Readers are advised, however, to check the product information sheet included in the package of each drug they plan to administer to be certain that changes have not been made in the recommended dose or in the contraindications for administration. This recommendation is of particular importance in regard to new or infrequently used drugs.

Fourth edition

Mosby-Year Book, Inc.
11830 Westline Industrial Drive, St. Louis, Missouri 63146

Library of Congress Cataloging in Publication Data

Brown, Meta.
    Drug calculations / Meta Brown, Joyce L. Mulholland. —4th ed.
      p.   cm.
    Includes index.
    ISBN 0-8016-6430-6
    1. Pharmaceutical arithmetic—Problems, exercises, etc.
  I. Mulholland, Joyce L. II. Title.
    [DNLM: 1. Drugs—administration & dosage—programmed instructions.
  QV 18 B879b]
  RS57.B76 1992
  615′.14—dc20
  DNLM/DLC
  for Library of Congress
                                                91-25664
                                               CIP

TS/DC 9 8 7 6 5 4 3 2

PREFACE

This workbook provides all the information, explanation, and practice needed to competently and confidently calculate medication dosages. Because the logical, step-by-step format is easy to understand, students can use the book for independent study or as part of a class. Graduates may find it useful in reviewing for licensure exams, and new practitioners will appreciate its value as a handy reference.

In this fourth edition, we have focused on meeting two goals: (1) to provide an instructionally sound text to ensure that all learners can readily master the material presented, and (2) to include all the information that is essential to safe, accurate drug calculation in current clinical practice.

Learning Aids

Each chapter begins with objectives that prepare students for the content to be covered and assist them in evaluating their mastery of that content. Explanations are clear and concise and include examples and illustrations to ensure student comprehension. Important rules are highlighted for emphasis and easy retrieval. Each section is followed by a series of practice problems to reinforce and evaluate learning. Problems move from simple to complex so that students can build on what they have learned. Each chapter ends with a test covering all material presented.

All problems have been updated to delete medications no longer used and to include new, commonly prescribed drugs. To help students prepare for what they will encounter in practice, numerous reproductions of drug labels and illustrations of syringes accompany the problems.

The ratio and proportion method is used throughout to provide a logical, accurate, and consistent means of calculation. This method also permits students to easily check their calculations. The answer key at the end of the book shows how to work out each problem, step-by-step, as well as how to verify the answer. This helps students identify specific errors in their calculations and encourages them to make a habit of checking their work. Because the book's pages are perforated for easy removal, students can compare their work side-by-side with the solution. A comprehensive examination provides additional practice and serves as an overall evaluation of learning.

Current and Comprehensive

For those who may be unsure of their mastery of basic math, a pretest is provided to evaluate knowledge and identify specific weaknesses. Chapter 1 reviews general mathematics so students can be confident in their abilities before moving on to drug calculations. Methods of rounding are included to help students calculate quickly and accurately.

Chapter 2 explains the ratio and proportion method and shows how to use it in calculating drug doses. Chapters 3 and 4 discuss the metric and apothecary systems and how to convert from one to the other as well as within systems. The metric system is stressed because of its wide use in health care. Chapter 5 deals with preparing medications from powders and crystals and determining the proper dilution strength.

Chapters 6 through 10 prepare the student to calculate dosages of various drugs in various settings. Each of these chapters include sample charting to emphasize the importance of maintaining current and accurate medication administration records. Chapter 6 introduces basic intravenous calculations and has been expanded to include piggyback administration. Chapter 7 discusses types of insulin, the special syringes used, and the calculation of dosages. Chapter 8 deals with heparin administration, and Chapter 9 highlights the special procedures used to calculate dosages for children. More complex IV titrations are presented in Chapter 10, which features a simplified method for calculating IV titrations in critical care settings. For those institutions where the nurse may still be responsible for preparing solutions, Chapter 11 provides guidelines.

Acknowledgments

We wish to thank Betty Gahart for allowing us to quote safe ranges of intravenous medications from her book, *Intravenous Medications*. We are also grateful to Medical Economics, publisher of the Physicians' Desk Reference, for permission to quote medication dosage ranges. Special thanks go to Carol Moore, R.N., M.N., Hutchinson Community Junior College, Hutchinson, Kansas and Jeanette Kowalski, R.N., M.S.N. Utilization Manager, St. Louis University Hospital, St. Louis, Missouri, who carefully reviewed the material in this book.

Meta Brown
Joyce L. Mulholland

CONTENTS

General mathematics pretest

Directions: Take this test completely. Then check your answers on page 179 to see which areas you may need to review.

Change to whole or mixed numbers:

1. $^{25}\!/_4$

2. $^{36}\!/_7$

Change to improper fractions:

3. $4^2\!/_9$

4. $9^1\!/_2$

Find the lowest common denominator (bottom number) in the following fractions:

5. $^4\!/_{11}$ and $^1\!/_6$

6. $^2\!/_5$ and $^5\!/_9$

Add the following numbers:

7. $^1\!/_5$, $^1\!/_6$, and $^2\!/_3$

8. $1^1\!/_2 + 3^1\!/_8 + 2^1\!/_6$

Subtract the following:

9. $^5\!/_7 - ^1\!/_4$

10. $8^1\!/_4 - 3^3\!/_8$

Multiply the following:

11. $^1\!/_6 \times ^1\!/_2$

12. $^2\!/_8 \times 1^1\!/_3$

Divide the following:

13. $^1\!/_3 \div ^2\!/_5$

14. $1^1\!/_8 \div 2^1\!/_2$

Express the following fractions reduced to lowest terms (numbers):

15. $^3\!/_{150}$

16. $^4\!/_{19}$

Write the following as decimals:

17. Fourteen hundredths

18. Three and sixteen thousandths

Add the following:

19. 3.04 + 1.865

20. 25.7 + 3.008

Subtract the following:

21. 3 − 0.04

22. 0.96 − 0.1359

Multiply the following:

23. 0.003 × 1.2

24. 3 × 0.5

Divide the following and carry to the third decimal place:

25. 201.1 ÷ 20

26. 20.6 ÷ 0.21

Change the following to decimals:

27. $^{23}/_{43}$

28. 9⅛

Solve the following percents:

29. 15% of 63

30. 1¾% of 4210

Change the following decimals to fractions:

31. 0.70

32. 0.492

33. Write 17% as a decimal and as a fraction.

34. Write ⅛ as a decimal and as a percent.

35. Write 0.014 as a fraction and as a percent.

CHAPTER 1

General mathematics

Objectives

- Convert fractions into whole and mixed numbers.
- Change mixed numbers into improper fractions.
- Find lowest common denominators in fractions.
- Add fractions and mixed numbers and reduce to lowest terms (reduce fractions).
- Subtract fractions and mixed numbers.
- Multiply fractions and mixed numbers.
- Divide fractions and mixed numbers.
- Given two fractions, determine which is greater and which is smaller.
- Distinguish among decimal fractions in tenths, hundredths, ten-thousandths, and hundred-thousandths.
- Read whole numbers and decimal fractions.
- Divide decimals to third decimal place.
- Add, subtract, and divide decimals.
- Change decimals to fractions.
- Reduce fractions to lowest terms.
- Change fractions to decimals.
- Change percent to fraction.
- Round decimals to the nearest tenth, hundredth, and whole number.
- Convert fraction to decimal.
- Change percent to decimal.
- Convert decimal to percent.
- Find percent.

A fraction is part of a whole number. The fraction ⅝ means that there are 8 parts to the whole number (bottom) but you want to measure only 6 of those parts (top number).

⅝ can be reduced by division of both the numbers by 2.

$$\frac{6 \div 2}{8 \div 2} = \frac{3}{4}$$

Changing improper fractions into whole or mixed numbers

An improper fraction has a large numerator and a small denominator, such as $^8/_4$.

RULES: **1** When the top number is larger than the bottom number, divide the bottom number into the top number.
2 Write the remainder as a fraction and reduce to lowest terms.

EXAMPLE: $^8/_4 = 8 \div 4 = 2$ *Whole number*

$^{16}/_6 = 16 \div 6 = 2^4/_6 = 2^2/_3$ *This is a mixed number* because it has a whole number plus a fraction.

1A ## Worksheet   (Answers on p. 180)

Change the following to whole numbers or mixed fractions:

1. $^8/_8 =$ 5. $^{34}/_6 =$ 8. $^{120}/_{64} =$

2. $^{13}/_4 =$ 6. $^{100}/_{25} =$ 9. $^{12}/_4 =$

3. $^6/_2 =$ 7. $^7/_4 =$ 10. $^{41}/_6 =$

4. $^{14}/_9 =$

Changing mixed numbers into improper fractions

> **RULES:**
> **1** Multiply the whole number by the bottom number of the fraction.
> **2** Add this to the top number of the fraction.
> **3** Write the sum as the top number of the fraction; the bottom number of the fraction remains the same.

EXAMPLE: $2\frac{3}{8} = \dfrac{8 \times 2 + 3}{8} = {}^{19}\!/_8$

$4\frac{2}{5} = \dfrac{20 + 2}{5} = {}^{22}\!/_5$

1B Worksheet   (Answers on p. 180)

Change the following to improper fractions:

1. $1\frac{1}{5} =$

2. $1\frac{1}{4} =$

3. $16\frac{1}{3} =$

4. $3\frac{7}{12} =$

5. $13\frac{3}{5} =$

6. $4\frac{3}{8} =$

7. $3\frac{5}{6} =$

8. $2\frac{5}{8} =$

9. $10\frac{3}{6} =$

10. $125\frac{2}{3} =$

Addition of fractions and mixed numbers

Finding lowest common denominator (in fraction)

RULES:	**1** Find the lowest common number that the bottom numbers can be divided into. **2** Change the fractions to equivalent fractions using these bottom numbers.

EXAMPLE: $2/3 = 16/24$
$7/8 = 21/24$
$1/6 = 4/24$

Addition of fractions and mixed numbers

RULE:	If fractions have the same bottom number, add the top numbers, write over the bottom number, and reduce.

EXAMPLE:

$$\frac{1}{5}$$
$$+\frac{2}{5}$$
$$\frac{3}{5}$$

RULE:	If fractions have different bottom numbers, find the lowest common number and then add the top numbers.

EXAMPLE:

$$\frac{3}{5} = \frac{9}{15}$$
$$+\frac{2}{3} = +\frac{10}{15}$$
$$\frac{19}{15} = 19 \div 15 = 1\,4/15$$

RULE:	To add mixed numbers, first add the fractions and then add this to the sum of the whole numbers.

EXAMPLE:

$$9^5/8 = 9^{15}/24$$
$$+6^1/6 = 6\ ^4/24$$
$$15^{19}/24$$

Worksheet (Answers on p. 180)

Add the following fractions and mixed numbers:

1. $\frac{1}{5}$
       $+\frac{2}{5}$

6. $\frac{1}{8}$
       $\frac{1}{4}$
      $+\frac{2}{9}$

2. $\frac{3}{5}$
       $+\frac{2}{3}$

7. $\frac{7}{9}$
       $\frac{4}{5}$
      $+\frac{9}{10}$

3. $6\frac{1}{6}$
      $+9\frac{5}{8}$

8. $3\frac{1}{4}$
      $+9\frac{3}{4}$

4. $1\frac{3}{8}$
      $+9\frac{9}{10}$

9. $8\frac{2}{5}$
      $14\frac{7}{10}$
      $+9\frac{9}{10}$

5. $2\frac{1}{4}$
      $+3\frac{1}{8}$

10. $2\frac{1}{3}$
       $4\frac{1}{6}$

Subtraction of fractions and mixed numbers

EXAMPLE: $27/32$ Difference between the top numbers (27 minus 18)
            $-18/32$ equals 9. Bottom number is 32.
            $9/32$

EXAMPLE: $7/8 = 21/24$ Difference between the top numbers (21 minus 16)
            $-2/3 = 16/24$ equals 5. Bottom number is 24.
            $5/24$

EXAMPLE: $21\ 7/16$ You cannot subtract the top numbers because 12 is
            $-\ 7\,12/16$ larger than 7. Therefore, you must make a whole
                        number out of $7/16$ and add the 7.

$$16/16 + 7/16 = 23/16$$

Because we added a whole number to the fraction, we must take a whole number away from 21 and make it 20. The problem now is set up as follows:

$$21\,7/16 = 20\,16/16 + 7/16 = \quad 20\,23/16$$
$$-\ \ 7\,12/16$$
$$13\,11/16$$

Worksheet   (Answers on p. 181)

Subtract fractions and mixed numbers (reduce answer to lowest terms):

1. $4/5$
    $-1/2$

6. $7/8$
    $-2/3$

2. $7^{16}/_{24}$
    $-3\ 1/8$

7. $3^5/_8$
    $-1^3/_8$

3. $21\ ^7/_{16}$
    $-\ \ 7^{12}/_{16}$

8. $5^3/_7$
    $-1^6/_7$

4. $27/_{32}$
    $-^{18}/_{32}$

9. 7
    $-1^3/_4$

5. $6^3/_{10}$
    $-2^1/_5$

10. $2^7/_8$
     $-\ \ ^3/_4$

Multiplication of fractions and mixed numbers

RULES:
1 Change mixed number to improper fraction.
2 Cancel if possible by dividing any top and bottom number by the largest number contained in each.
3 Multiply remaining top number to find top-number result.
4 Multiply bottom number to find bottom-number result.
5 Reduce answer to lowest terms.

EXAMPLE:

1 $\quad \frac{4}{5} \times \frac{15}{16} = \frac{\overset{1}{\cancel{4}}}{\underset{1}{\cancel{5}}} \times \frac{\overset{3}{\cancel{15}}}{\underset{4}{\cancel{16}}} = \frac{3}{4}$

2 $\quad 4\frac{1}{2} \times 2\frac{1}{4} = \frac{9}{2} \times \frac{9}{4} = \frac{81}{8} = 10\frac{1}{8}$

3 $\quad 6 \times \frac{3}{8} = \frac{6}{1} \times \frac{3}{8} = \frac{\overset{3}{\cancel{6}}}{1} \times \frac{3}{\underset{4}{\cancel{8}}} = \frac{9}{4} = 2\frac{1}{4}$

1E Worksheet (Answers on p. 182)

Multiply the following fractions and mixed numbers (reduce answer to lowest terms):

1. $\frac{1}{3} \times \frac{2}{4} =$

2. $5\frac{1}{2} \times 3\frac{1}{8} =$

3. $1\frac{3}{4} \times 3\frac{1}{7} =$

4. $4 \times 3\frac{1}{8} =$

5. $\frac{2}{4} \times 2\frac{1}{6} =$

6. $\frac{1}{5} \times \frac{1}{3} =$

7. $\frac{3}{4} \times \frac{5}{8} =$

8. $\frac{5}{6} \times 1\frac{9}{16} =$

9. $\frac{5}{100} \times 900 =$

10. $2\frac{1}{10} \times 4\frac{1}{3} =$

Division of fractions and mixed numbers

> **RULES:**
> 1 Change mixed number to improper fractions.
> 2 Turn the number after the ÷ (division) sign upside down.
> 3 Follow steps for multiplying and reduce any fractions.

EXAMPLE:

$$1 \quad \frac{1}{2} \div \frac{5}{8} = \frac{1}{2} \times \frac{8}{5} = \frac{8}{10} = \frac{4}{5}$$

$$2 \quad 8\frac{3}{4} \div 15 = \frac{35}{4} \times \frac{1}{15} = \frac{\overset{7}{\cancel{35}}}{4} \times \frac{1}{\underset{3}{\cancel{15}}} = \frac{7}{12}$$

1F ## Worksheet   (Answers on p. 182)

Divide the following fractions and mixed numbers:

1. ²⁄₅ ÷ ⅝ =

2. 8¾ ÷ 15 =

3. ¾ ÷ ⅛ =

4. ¹⁄₁₆ ÷ ¼ =

5. ⅓ ÷ ½ =

6. ¾ ÷ 6 =

7. 2 ÷ ⅕ =

8. 3⅜ ÷ 4½ =

9. ⅗ ÷ ⅜ =

10. 4 ÷ 2⅛ =

Value of fractions

> **RULE:** The smaller the bottom number of a fraction, the greater it is in value. Make a whole number out of a fraction to see which one is larger.

EXAMPLE: ⅙ is greater than ⅑ because the bottom number is smaller.

> **RULE:** To make a whole number out of the fraction ⁶⁄₆ means there are 6 parts to the whole number.

EXAMPLE:

$\frac{1}{6}$	$\frac{1}{6}$	$\frac{1}{6}$	$\frac{1}{6}$	$\frac{1}{6}$	$\frac{1}{6}$

= 6 parts   Each ⅙ part is larger than the ⅑ part.

$\frac{1}{9}$	$\frac{1}{9}$	$\frac{1}{9}$	$\frac{1}{9}$	$\frac{1}{9}$	$\frac{1}{9}$	$\frac{1}{9}$	$\frac{1}{9}$	$\frac{1}{9}$

= 9 parts   Each ⅑ part is smaller than the ⅙ part.

Which would you rather have: $\frac{1}{6}$ or $\frac{1}{9}$ of your favorite pie?

1G Worksheet   (Answers on p. 183)

Solve the following problems:

1. Which is greater: ⅓ or ⅕?

2. Which is smaller: ¹⁄₁₀₀ or ¹⁄₁₅₀?

3. Which is greater: ¹⁄₂₅₀ or ¹⁄₃₀₀?

4. Which is smaller: ⅙ or ⅛?

In the following problems, *estimate* answers before beginning. This is a good habit to develop.

5. Doctor ordered gr $\frac{1}{150}$. On hand you have gr $\frac{1}{200}$ tablets. Will you need to give more or less than what is on hand?

6. On hand you have gr $\frac{1}{150}$ tablets. Doctor ordered gr $\frac{1}{300}$. Will you need to give more or less than what is on hand?

7. Doctor ordered gr $\frac{1}{6}$. You have on hand gr $\frac{1}{4}$ tablets. Will you need more or less than what is on hand?

8. Doctor ordered gr $\frac{1}{10}$. On hand you have gr $\frac{1}{4}$ tablets. Will you need to give more or less than what is on hand?

9. On hand you have gr $\frac{1}{200}$. Doctor ordered gr $\frac{1}{100}$. Will you need to give more or less than what is on hand?

10. Doctor ordered gr $\frac{1}{8}$. On hand you have gr $\frac{1}{6}$ tablets. Will you need to give more or less than what is on hand?

Value of decimals

A decimal fraction is a fraction whose denominator (bottom number) is 10, 100, 1000, 10,000, and so on. It differs from a common fraction in that the denominator (bottom number) is *not* written but is expressed by the proper placement of the decimal point.

Observe the scale below. All whole numbers are to the left of the decimal point; all decimal fractions are to the right.

RULES: 1 All whole numbers are to the left of the decimal; all decimal fractions are to the right of the decimal point.
2 To read a decimal fraction, read the number to the right of the decimal and use the name that applies to "place value" of the *last* figure. All decimal fractions read with a *ths* on the end, except *half* and *thirds*.

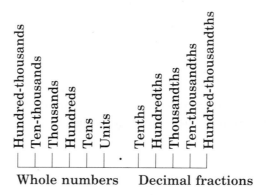

Whole numbers   Decimal fractions

EXAMPLE: 0.257 = Two-hundred-fifty-seven thousand*ths*
0.2057 = Two-thousand-fifty-seven ten-thousand*ths*
0.20057 = Twenty-thousand-fifty-seven hundred-thousand*ths*

RULE: To read a whole number and a fraction, the decimal point reads as an *and.*

EXAMPLE: 327.006 = Three hundred twenty-seven *and* six thousand*ths*

Worksheet   (Answers on p. 183)

Read the following out loud:

1.	0.08	3.	0.0017	5.	0.0006
2.	0.092	4.	3287.467	6.	100.01

Express the following as decimal fractions:

7. Thirty-six hundredths _____

8. Three thousandths _____

9. Eight ten-thousandths _____

10. Two and seventeen thousandths _____

11. Five hundredths _____

12. Four and one tenth _____

13. Twenty-four and two tenths _____

14. Fifteen and one hundredth _____

15. Nine and two ten-thousandths _____

16. Three and eight thousandths _____

17. One hundred and eighteen thousandths _____

18. Eighteen and fifteen hundredths _____

19. Fifty-five thousandths _____

20. Thirty-four and one tenth _____

Division of decimals

EXAMPLE:

$$15 \div 6.2 = 6.2\overline{)15.0,000}$$

$$
\begin{array}{r}
2.419 \\
6.2\,)\overline{15.0,000} \\
12\ 4 \\
\hline
2\ 6\ 0 \\
2\ 4\ 8 \\
\hline
1\ 20 \\
62 \\
\hline
580 \\
558 \\
\hline
22
\end{array}
$$

Worksheet   (Answers on p. 184)

Divide the following and carry to the *third* decimal place if necessary:

1.   158.4 ÷ 48

2.   200 ÷ 6.0

3.   15.06 ÷ 6

4.   79.4 ÷ 0.87

5.   670.8 ÷ 0.78

6.   78.6 ÷ 2.43

7.   26.78 ÷ 8.2

8.   266.5 ÷ 5.78

9.   10.80 ÷ 6.5

10.   76.53 ÷ 10

Addition of decimals

EXAMPLE:

$$0.8 \qquad 3.27$$
$$+0.5 \qquad +0.06$$
$$\overline{1.3} \qquad \overline{3.33}$$

REMEMBER: Line up the decimal points.

1J # Worksheet   (Answers on p. 185)

Add the following decimals:

1. $0.8 + 0.5 =$

2. $3.27 + 0.06 + 2 =$

3. $5.01 + 2.999 =$

4. $15.6 + 0.19 + 200 =$

5. $210.79 + 2 + 68.4 =$

6. $88.6 + 576.46 + 79.0 =$

7. $6.77 + 102 + 88.3 =$

8. $79.4 + 68.44 + 3.00 =$

9. $10.56 + 356.4 =$

10. $99.7 + 293.23 =$

Multiplication of decimals

EXAMPLE: $2.6 \times 0.0002 =$ 2.6 (1 decimal place)
$\times 0.0002$ (4 decimal places)
0.00052 (5 decimal places starting at the right in the answer)

1K Worksheet   (Answers on p. 185)

Multiply the following decimals:

1. $3.14 \times 0.002 =$

2. $95.26 \times 1.125 =$

3. $100 \times 0.5 =$

4. $2.14 \times 0.03 =$

5. $36.8 \times 70.1 =$

6. $203.7 \times 28 =$

7. $88 \times 90.1 =$

8. $2.76 \times 0.003 =$

9. $54.5 \times 21 =$

10. $200 \times 0.2 =$

Subtraction of decimals

> **RULES:**
> 1 Write decimals in a column, keeping the decimal points under each other.
> 2 Subtract as in whole numbers.
> 3 Place the decimal point in the answer directly under the decimal point in the sums to be added (zeros can be added *after* the decimal point without changing the value).

EXAMPLE: $0.6 - 0.524 =$

$$\begin{array}{r} 0.600 \\ -0.524 \\ \hline 0.076 \end{array}$$

REMEMBER: Line up the decimal points.

1L Worksheet   (Answers on p. 186)

Subtract the following decimals:

1. $98.4 - 66.50 =$

2. $108.56 - 5.40 =$

3. $0.450 - 0.367 =$

4. $21.78 - 19.88 =$

5. $266.44 - 0.56 =$

6. $7.066 - 0.200 =$

7. $34.678 - 0.502 =$

8. $78.567 - 6.77 =$

9. $1.723 - 0.683 =$

10. $0.8100 - 0.6701 =$

Changing decimals to fractions

RULES:
1. The numbers to the *right* of the decimal can be written as a fraction because they are only part of the whole number.
2. REMEMBER: The first number past the decimal to the *right* is ten*ths* (10), the second is hundred*ths* (100), the third is thousand*ths* (1000), the fourth is ten-thousand*ths* (10,000), and so on.
3. So if your problem has 3 numbers to the *right* of the decimal, just remove the decimal and put the number over 1000.

EXAMPLES:
1. 0.375 has 3 numbers to the *right* of the decimal. To make a fraction out of 0.375 and also get rid of the decimal, just put it over 1000.

   0.375 written as a fraction is $375/1000$.

   It's easy to remember: 3 numbers on top and 3 zeros on the bottom.
2. 0.91 written as a fraction is $91/100$.

   The idea is the same as above: 2 numbers on top and 2 zeros on the bottom.

Worksheet   (Answers on p. 186)

Change decimals to fractions and reduce to lowest terms:

1. 0.4 =

2. 0.8 =

3. 0.25 =

4. 4.08 =

5. 1.32 =

6. 0.5 =

7. 0.75 =

8. 0.2 =

9. 0.65 =

10. 0.7 =

Changing common fractions to decimals

> **RULE:** Divide the top number by the bottom number and place the decimal point in the proper position.

$$
\text{EXAMPLE:} \quad \frac{2}{5} = 5\overline{)2.00} \quad \begin{array}{l} 0.40 = 0.4 \\ \underline{2.0} \\ 0 \end{array}
$$

1N Worksheet (Answers on p. 187)

Carry out division to *third* decimal place:

1. $\frac{19}{100} =$

2. $\frac{9}{7} =$

3. $5\frac{9}{16} =$

4. $\frac{1}{5} =$

5. $\frac{2}{3} =$

6. $\frac{1}{2} =$

7. $\frac{1}{12} =$

8. $\frac{6}{8} =$

9. $\frac{15}{200} =$

10. $\frac{20}{8} =$

Rounding decimals

RULES:	**1** Calculate *one* decimal place beyond the desired place.		
	2 If the final digit is 4 or less, make no adjustment. If the final digit is 5 or more, *increase* the prior digit by one number.		
	3 Drop the final digit.		

EXAMPLE:

1 Round 2.7 to the nearest whole number. Examine the tenths column.
Because .7 is more than 5, the answer is 3 and .7 is dropped.

2 Round 2.58 to the nearest tenth.
Calculate to the second decimal place (hundredths column) and examine it.
Because .8 is more than 5, round 2.58 to 2.6.
Drop the 8.

3 Round 3.763 to the nearest hundredth.
Calculate to the third decimal place (thousandths column) and examine it.
Because 3 is less than 5, no adjustment will be made in the hundredths column and the 3 is dropped.
The answer is 3.76.

MORE EXAMPLES:

	Nearest whole number	Nearest tenth	Nearest hundredth
1.689	2	1.7	1.69
204.534	205	204.5	204.53
7.87	8	7.9	7.87
3.366	3	3.4	3.37
0.845*	1	0.8	0.85

*To reduce reading errors, develop the habit of placing a 0 (zero) in front of decimals when a whole number is absent.

Worksheet (Answers on p. 188)

Round the decimal to the nearest whole number, the nearest tenth, and the nearest hundredth:

		Nearest whole number	Nearest tenth	Nearest hundredth
1.	93.489	_____	_____	_____
2.	25.430	_____	_____	_____
3.	38.10	_____	_____	_____
4.	57.8888	_____	_____	_____
5.	0.0092	_____	_____	_____
6.	3.144	_____	_____	_____
7.	8.999	_____	_____	_____
8.	77.788	_____	_____	_____
9.	12.959	_____	_____	_____
10.	5.7703	_____	_____	_____

Worksheet (Answers on p. 188)

Round your answers to the problems below to the nearest whole number, the nearest tenth, and the nearest hundredth:

		Nearest whole number	Nearest tenth	Nearest hundredth
1.	$25.3 \times 4.2 =$	_____	_____	_____
2.	$9.3 \times 2.86 =$	_____	_____	_____
3.	$4.5 \times 7.57 =$	_____	_____	_____
4.	$1.3 \times 9.69 =$	_____	_____	_____
5.	$2.4 \times 5.88 =$	_____	_____	_____
6.	$8 \div 5 =$	_____	_____	_____
7.	$4.1 \div 3 =$	_____	_____	_____
8.	$5 \div 1.2 =$	_____	_____	_____
9.	$9 \div 2.2 =$	_____	_____	_____
10.	$10.2 \div 3 =$	_____	_____	_____

Percentages, decimals, and fractions

The term *percent* and its symbol (%) mean hundred*ths*. A percent number is a fraction whose top number is already known and whose bottom is *always* understood to be 100.

Changing a percent to a fraction

RULE: The top number is the percent and the bottom number is always 100.

EXAMPLE: 1 5% written as a fraction is $5/100$.

Drop the percent sign when converting 5% to $5/100$.

2 $\frac{1}{2}$% is written as a fraction $\dfrac{1/2}{100}$. You cannot leave the problem like this. $\dfrac{1/2}{100}$ means $1/2 \div 100 = 1/2 \times 1/100 = 1/200$. The problem is completed when $\dfrac{1/2}{100} = 1/2 \times 1/100 = 1/200$.

Converting a fraction to a decimal

RULE: The fraction $5/100$ can be made into a decimal by dividing the bottom number into the top number.

EXAMPLE: 1 To change $5/100$ into a decimal means $5 \div 100$.

$$100)\overline{5.00}^{\,.05} \qquad \text{Don't forget the decimal point.}$$
$$\underline{5\ 00}$$

2 Change $1/200$ to a decimal. Divide the bottom number into the top number.

$$1 \div 200 = 200)\overline{1.000}^{\,.005}$$
$$\underline{1\ 000}$$

Changing a percent to a decimal

A percent number can be changed to a decimal by having its decimal point moved 2 places to the *left* to signify hundred*ths.*

EXAMPLE: 1 5% written as a decimal is 0.05.
REMEMBER: Move the decimal 2 places to the *left* and drop the % sign.
2 0.5% written as a decimal is 0.005.
REMEMBER: Move the decimal 2 places to the *left* and drop the % sign.

Converting a decimal to a percent

RULE: The only thing you must do is to move the decimal point 2 places to the *right* and add the percent sign.

EXAMPLE: 1 0.05 is a decimal. To make it a percent, move the decimal point 2 places to the *right* and add the % sign. Therefore 0.05 = 5%.
2 0.005 = 0.5% or ½%

Worksheet (Answers on p. 188)

	Fraction	Decimal	Percent
1.	_____	_____	66⅔%
2.	½	_____	_____
3.	_____	_____	6.5%
4.	1/12	_____	_____
5.	3/1000	_____	_____
6.	_____	0.10	_____
7.	_____	_____	250%
8.	_____	0.35	_____
9.	4/5	_____	_____
10.	_____	_____	78%

If you are having difficulty with fractions, decimals, or percents, review this chapter or see your instructor.

Finding the percentage

EXAMPLE: 23% of $64 = 64 \times 0.23 = 14.72$

1R Worksheet (Answers on p. 189)

1. 114% of $240 =$

2. 2% of $1500 =$

3. $\frac{1}{2}\%$ of $9328 =$

4. $\frac{1}{3}\%$ of $930 =$

5. 28% of $50 =$

6. 9% of $200 =$

7. 120% of $400 =$

8. 5% of $105.80 =$

9. 10% of $520 =$

10. 3% of $40.80 =$

■ General Mathematics Test (Answers on p. 190)

Change to whole or mixed numbers:

1. $^{34}/_6$ 2. $^{48}/_7$

Change to improper fractions:

3. $13^3/_5$ 4. $3^5/_6$

Find the lowest common bottom number in the following fractions:

5. $^{17}/_{20}$ and $^4/_5$ 6. $^7/_8$ and $^3/_5$

Add the following numbers:

7. $^1/_{18}$, $^1/_4$, and $^2/_9$ 8. $5^1/_8$, $1^1/_4$, and $4^1/_2$

Subtract the following:

9. $^7/_8 - ^2/_3$ 10. $6^2/_4 - 5^1/_2$

Multiply the following:

11. $^1/_5 \times ^1/_3$ 12. $^5/_6 \times ^2/_8$

Divide the following:

13. $^3/_4 \div ^1/_8$ 14. $3^3/_8 \div 4^1/_2$

Express the following ratios as fractions reduced to lowest terms (numbers):

15. 2:500   16. 2:13

Write the following as decimals:

17. Thirty-six hundredths _____   18. Two and seventeen thousandths _____

Add the following:

19. 5.01 + 2.999

20. 36.87 + 8.26 + 15.84

Subtract the following:

21. 4 − 0.176

22. 0.41 − 0.2538

Multiply the following:

23. 0.0005 × 0.02

24. 5 × 0.7

Divide the following and carry to the third decimal place:

25. 158.4 ÷ 48

26. 79.4 ÷ 0.87

Change the following to decimals:

27. $^{57}/_{48}$

28. 8$^1/_{16}$

Solve the following percents:

29. 24% of 52

30. 6$^1/_4$% of 9328

Change the following decimals to fractions:

31. 0.400

32. 0.285

33. Write 43% as a decimal and as a fraction.

34. Write $^1/_{10}$ as a decimal and as a percent.

35. Write 0.029 as a fraction and as a percent.

36. Round 8.876 to the nearest tenth.

37. Round 1.346 to the nearest hundredth.

38. Round 4.8 to the nearest whole number.

39. Round 70.298 to the nearest whole number.

40. Round 0.065 to the nearest hundredth.

CHAPTER 2

Ratio and proportion

Objectives

- Express ratios as fractions.
- Reduce fractions to lowest numerical terms.
- Solve ratio/proportion problems for x.
- Solve verbal and numerical ratio/proportion problems for x.
- Solve one-step ratio/proportion problems.
- Estimate answers.
- Prove answers.

Ratio

> **RULE:** A ratio indicates the relationship of one quantity to another. It indicates *division* and may be expressed in fraction form.

EXAMPLE: ⅓ may be expressed as a ratio 1:3.

2A Worksheet (Answers on p. 190)

Express the following ratios as fractions reduced to lowest terms:

1. 2:4	5. 43:86	8. 1:5
2. 4:6	6. 2:13	9. 1:150
3. 2:500	7. 7:49	10. 4:100
4. 6:1000		

Proportion

A proportion shows the relationship between two equal ratios. A proportion may be expressed as 3:5::6:10 or 3:5 = 6:10.

To solve the ratio and proportion problems, just do this:

> **RULES:**
> **1** Multiply the two inside numbers.
> **2** Multiply the two outside numbers.
> **3** The answers should be the same.

EXAMPLE: 3:5::6:10
multiply

Multiply the two *inside* numbers: 5 × 6 = 30
Multiply the two *outside* numbers: 3 × 10 = 30

How to solve the problem when one of the numbers is unknown or x

Multiply the x first and put it on the *left* side of the equation.

EXAMPLE: 3:5::x:10

Multiply inside numbers: $5x$. Multiply outside numbers: 3 × 10 = 30. The equation will now look like this: $5x = 30$.

Now you must get x to stand alone. Cancel it out, and you will never go wrong. Whatever you do to one side you must do to the other to keep them equal. Canceling out eliminates the chance of dividing the wrong sides into each other. The end product of canceling out is a fraction, that is ³⁰⁄₅.
A fraction means that the bottom number is always divided into the top number.

EXAMPLE: This cancels the 5 out: $\dfrac{\cancel{5}x}{\cancel{5}} = \dfrac{30}{5}$

The only part of the problem left unsolved is ³⁰⁄₅. As you know, ³⁰⁄₅ means 30 ÷ 5 = 6; so $x = 6$.

Put the entire problem together, following the five steps outlined above. Remember to always put x on the *left*-hand side.

multiply
3:5::x:10   or $\dfrac{3}{5} \times \dfrac{x}{10}$
multiply

$5x = 30$ $5x = 30$

What you do to one side of the equation you must do to the other. This cancels out the 5 and leaves x.

$$\frac{\cancel{5}x}{\cancel{5}} = \frac{30}{5} \qquad \text{This means } 30 \div 5 \text{ or } 5\overline{)30}$$

$$x = 6 \qquad\qquad\qquad\qquad\qquad \begin{array}{r} 6 \\ \underline{30} \\ 0 \end{array}$$

How do you know your answer is correct?

To *prove* your answer, just substitute the answer for the x in the problem, multiply the inside numbers together, and then multiply the outside numbers together.

EXAMPLE: PROOF: 3:5::6:10

$$5 \times 6 = 30$$
$$3 \times 10 = 30$$

Now you are ready to solve for x.

2B Worksheet (Answers on p. 190)

Solve the following problems for x:

1. ½:x::1:8

2. 9:x::5:300

3. ¹⁄₁₀₀₀:¹⁄₁₀₀::x:60

4. ¼:500::x:1000

5. 36:12::¹⁄₁₀₀:x

6. 6:24::0.75:x

7. x:600::4:120

8. 0.7:70::x:1000

9. 9:27::300:x

10. 6:12::¼:x

Worksheet   (Answers on p. 192)

REMEMBER: Multiply two inside numbers, multiply two outside numbers, put x on the *left*.

Solve for x:

1. $\frac{1}{200} : x :: 1 : 800$

2. $15 : 30 :: x : 12$

3. $\frac{1}{1000} : \frac{1}{100} :: x : 30$

4. $6 : 12 :: 0.25 : x$

5. $300 : 5 :: x : \frac{1}{60}$

6. $\frac{1}{150} : \frac{1}{200} :: 2 : x$

7. $\frac{1}{2} : \frac{1}{6} :: \frac{1}{4} : x$

8. $7.5 : 12 :: x : 28$

9. $15 : x :: 1.5 : 10$

10. $10 : x :: 0.4 : 12$

Ratio and proportion: how to set up

EXAMPLE: Apples:*Pears*::Apples:*x Pears*

EXAMPLE: You wish to make a floral bouquet of 6 daffodils for every 4 roses. How many daffodils will you use for 30 roses?

Know   **Want to know**

6 daffodils:4 roses::*x* daffodils:30 roses   PROOF: $4 \times 45 = 180$

$$\frac{\cancel{4}x}{\cancel{4}} = \frac{180}{4} = 180 \div 4 = 45 \qquad\qquad 6 \times 30 = 180$$

Left
$4x = 180$

$x = 45$ daffodils

Worksheet   (Answers on p. 194)

Problems to set up and prove:

1. You have a recipe for cocoa—4 scoops make 6 cups of cocoa. You want to make 18 cups for a party. How many scoops of cocoa? Set up a proportion.

    $4:6 = x:18$

    $\dfrac{6x}{6} = \dfrac{72}{6} = 12$

2. You are making coffee, and 7 scoops make 8 cups. How many scoops make 40 cups?

    $7:8 = x:40$

    $7 \times 40 = 280$ $\dfrac{8x}{8} = \dfrac{280}{8} = x = 35$

    $x = 35$

3. You have to make a fruit basket with 6 bananas for every 9 apples. How many bananas for 72 apples?

    $6:9 = x:72$

    $\dfrac{9x}{9} = \dfrac{432}{9} = 48$ $x = 48$ bananas

4. Doctor ordered 450 mg of aspirin. On hand you have 300 mg in 1 tablet. How many tablets will you give?

    $1:300 mg$ $x = 450 mg$

    $\dfrac{300x}{300} = \dfrac{450}{300}$ 1.50

5. You wish to plant 8 bushes for every 2 trees in your yard. How many bushes for 36 trees? (Estimate and prove.)

    $8:2 = x:36$

    $\dfrac{2x}{2} = \dfrac{288}{2} = x = 144$

6. Doctor ordered 4 cups of All-Bran every day. How many days would it take to consume 84 cups of All-Bran? (Estimate and prove.)

    $4 cups:1 = 84:x$

    $1:4 cup = x:84$

    $\dfrac{4x}{4} = \dfrac{84}{4} = x = 21$ days

7. It takes 4 cups of flour to make 3 loaves of bread. How many loaves of bread can be made from 24 cups of flour?

4 cups : 3 loaves = 24 cups x loaves

3:4 x loaves : 24
4x
3×24 = 72

$\frac{4x}{4} = \frac{72}{4}$ x = 4√72   18

8. Your recipe for punch calls for 3 cups of soda for every ½ cup of fruit juice. How many cups of soda will you need for 2 cups of fruit juice?

3 cups soda : .5 cups juice = x soda : 2 cups juice

.5x
6 cups.

$\frac{.5x}{.5} = \frac{6 cups}{.5}$ = x = 6.0   12 cups.

9. You need 4 tbsp of sugar for every glass of lemonade you prepare. How many tablespoons of sugar will you need for 6 glasses of lemonade?

4 tbsp sug : 1 glass = x sug : 6 glass

1x
24 glasses

$\frac{4x}{x} = \frac{24}{1}$ = 24

10. Doctor ordered 4 capsules every day. How many capsules would you need for 14 days?

4 capsules : 1 = x : 14

1x
56

$\frac{4x}{x} = \frac{56}{1}$ x = 56

Ratio and proportion: how to set up

EXAMPLE: Make a necklace that has 19 blue beads for every 1 yellow bead. How many blue beads are needed if you have 8 yellow beads?

(Prove your answer.)

Have   **Want to know**

19 blue beads:1 yellow bead::x blue beads:8 yellow beads

—— multiply ——

—— multiply ——

$1x = 152$ blue beads needed   PROOF: $19 \times 8 = 152$

$1 \times 152 = 152$

Worksheet   (Answers on p. 196)

Use ratio and proportion. Label and prove your answers.

1. The office needed 4000 envelopes. You have on hand boxes that contain 200 envelopes per box. How many boxes will you send?

200 env : 1 box = 4000 env ; x boxes

1 box : 200 env = x box : 4000 env.

$$\frac{200x}{4000}$$

$$\frac{200x}{200} = \frac{4000}{200} \qquad \frac{40}{2} = 20$$

2. Ordered are 300 computer disks. You have on hand packages that contain 10 disks per package. How many packages will you send?

10 disks : 1 pk = 300 dis = x pk

1 : 10 = x pk : 300 disk

$$\frac{10x}{300 disk}$$

$$\frac{10x}{10} = \frac{300 disk}{10} = x = 10\overline{)300} \quad \frac{30}{30}$$

3. If you have one computer allocated for every 18 students, how many computers will be needed for an enrollment of 1280 students?

1 : 18 stud = x : com : 1280 students

$$\frac{18x}{1280s}$$

$$\frac{18x}{18} = \frac{1280}{18}$$

70 Comp.

4. The doctor tells you to drink 3 glasses of H_2O and eat 2 apples every day. How many apples will you have eaten when you have drunk 24 glasses of water?

3 gl (W) : 2 app = 24 glasses : x

2 : 3 = x : 24 glass

$$\frac{3x}{48}$$

$$\frac{3x}{3} = \frac{48}{3} = 16$$

5. If you were going to give all the teachers 6 pens for every 8 pencils, how many pens would you give for 72 pencils?

6 pens : 8 pencils = x pens : 72 pencils

$$\frac{8x}{432}$$

$$\frac{8x}{8} = \frac{432}{8} = 8\overline{)432} \quad \frac{54}{40} \quad \frac{32}{32}$$

6. If you were making an omelet with ½ tsp of salt for every 3 eggs, how much salt would you use for 30 eggs?

½ tsp : 3 egg = x salt : 30 eggs

$$\frac{3x}{.5 \times 30}$$

$$\frac{3x}{3} = \frac{15}{3} = 5$$

7. If your coffeemaker makes 8 cups of coffee for every 7 scoops of coffee, how many scoops would you need to make 24 cups of coffee?

7 scoops : 8 cups = x scoops : 24 cups

$\frac{}{8x}$

7 × 24 = 168

$\frac{8x}{8} = \frac{168}{8} = 8\overline{)168}\ \ 21$

8. Your flower arrangements call for 5 carnations for each fern. How many carnations would you need to order for 10 ferns?

5 carn : 1 fern = x carn : 10 fern

$\frac{}{1x}$

5 × 10   50

$\frac{1x}{1} = \frac{50}{1}$

9. If you need 2 tbsp of vinegar for each cup of water, how many tablespoons would you need for 10 cups of water?

2 tbls = 1   = x tbls : 10 cups H_2O

$\frac{}{1x}$

2 × 10 = 20

$\frac{1x}{1} = \frac{20}{1}$ (20)

10. If you were using ½ cup of milk for every 3 cups of flour, how much milk would you need for 21 cups of flour?

.5 : 3 cups   x milk : 21 cups flour

$\frac{}{3x}$

.5 × 21 = $\frac{21.}{.5}$

10.5.

$\frac{3x}{3} = \frac{10.5}{3}$

$3\overline{)10.5}$ 3.5
9
15

Worksheet (Answers on p. 198)

Use ratio and proportion. Label and prove your answers.

1. Ordered are 120 centerpieces. They are delivered in units of 10 per carton. How many cartons will you receive?

    10 centerpieces : 1 carton = 120 cent = x

    1 : 10 cent = x = 120 cut $\frac{10x}{10}$ $\frac{120}{10}$ = 10⟌120

2. You have to take 4 tsp of medicine every day. The bottle contains 80 teaspoons. How many days will the bottle last?

    1 day : 4 tsp = x days : 80 tsp. $\frac{4x}{4} = \frac{80}{4} = 20$

3. If you need 10 diapers a day, how many days will a package of 50 diapers last?

    1 : 10 diapers = x days : 50 diap $\frac{10x}{10} = \frac{50}{10} = 5$

4. You are making 2-egg omelets. The recipe calls for 3 drops of Tabasco sauce for each omelet. If you use 12 eggs, how many drops of Tabasco sauce will you need?

    3 drops : 2 eggs = x drops : 12 eggs $\frac{2x}{2} = \frac{36}{2} = 18$

5. Each apartment has 1½ bathrooms. If there are 75 apartments, how many bathrooms are there? If you needed 3 towels for each bathroom, how many would you order?

    1.5 : 1 = x : 75 apt   112.5

    1.5 × 75 =   112.5 × 3 = 337.5 or 338

Worksheet (Answers on p. 199)

Use ratio and proportion. Label and prove your answers.

1. If each shelf holds 35 books, how many shelves will be needed for 280 books?

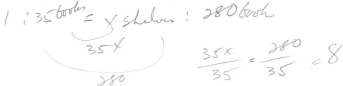

2. You're baking brownies. The recipe calls for 2 tbsp cocoa for each ½ cup of flour. How many tablespoons of cocoa will you need for 6 cups of flour?

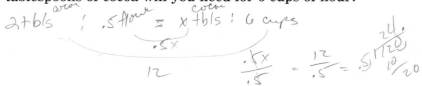

3. The computer can print 60 lines per page. How many pages will the manuscript be for 1800 typewritten lines?

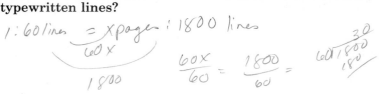

4. Your car gets an oil change every 2500 miles. How many oil changes will you have had when the odometer reads 100,000 miles?

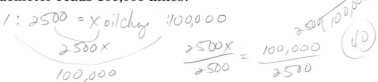

5. If you have 4 cookies for each 6 guests, how many cookies will you have available for 54 guests?

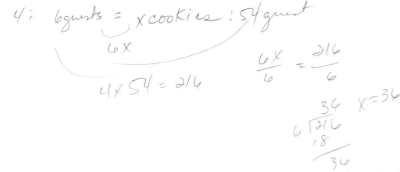

■ Ratio and Proportion Test (Answers on p. 200)

SHOW ALL WORK.
Solve the following proportions for x and prove your answers.

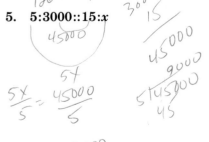

1. $9:x::5:300$

2. $6:24::0.75:x$

$6x = 24 \cdot .75$
$6x = 18$ $\dfrac{6x}{6} = $

3. $8:16::x:24$

$\dfrac{16x}{16} = \dfrac{192}{16} = x = \boxed{32}$

4. $x:600::4:120$

$\dfrac{120x}{120} = \dfrac{240}{120} = x = \boxed{2}$

5. $5:3000::15:x$

$\dfrac{5x}{5} = \dfrac{45000}{5}$

$y = 9000$

6. $0.7:70::x:1000$

$\dfrac{70x}{70} = \dfrac{7000}{70}$

$x = 100$

7. $9:27::300:x$

$\dfrac{9x}{9} = \dfrac{8100}{9} = x = \boxed{900}$

8. $6:12::\frac{1}{4}:x$

$\dfrac{6x}{6} = \dfrac{3}{6} = x = .5$

9. $25:x::75:3000$

$\dfrac{75x}{75} = \dfrac{75000}{75}$

$x = \boxed{1000}$

10. $0.6:10::0.5:x$

$\dfrac{.6x}{6} = \dfrac{5.0}{6}$

CHAPTER 3

Metric system

Objectives

- Convert milligrams, micrograms, grams, and kilograms.
- Memorize milliliter and liter conversions.
- Calculate gram and milligram conversion problems.
- Calculate one-step metric conversion problems by ratio and proportion method.
- Identify one- and two-step metric conversion problems.
- Calculate two-step metric conversion problems by ratio and proportion method.

Explanation

The metric system is now being used exclusively in the *United States Pharmacopeia* and before long will probably be the only system used in drug dosage. Arabic numbers and decimals are used with this system. Blame the French if you don't like the metric system, but it's really easier than any other method because it is a decimal system (based on the number 10) and all the math involved is done by moving decimals.

The basic metric units are multiplied and divided always by a multiple of 10 to form the entire system. (The period for abbreviation often may not appear in some writings.) There are only a few equivalents that are used in medicine. These are as follows:

MEMORIZE:

Weight

1 mg (milligram) = 1000 µg (or mcg) (micrograms)
1 g (gram) = 1000 mg (milligrams)
1 kg (kilogram) = 2.2 lb = 1000 g or Gm (grams)

Volume

1000 ml (milliliters) or cc (cubic centimeters) = 1 L (liter)

A milliliter (ml) is equivalent to a cubic centimeter (cc), and for all practical purposes these units may be used interchangeably. However, the use of milliliter is preferable. Hence:

$$1000 \text{ cc} = 1 \text{ L (liter)}$$
$$1000 \text{ ml} = 1 \text{ L (liter)}$$

PLEASE NOTE: The symbol, such as g or mg, always *follows* the amount.

EXAMPLE: 1000 mg
                    1 g

■ Metric measurements, prefixes, and their equivalents

Prefix	Numerical value	Power of base 10	Meaning
deci	.1	10^{-1}	Tenth part of
centi	.01	10^{-2}	Hundredth part of
milli	.001	10^{-3}	Thousandth part of
micro	.000001	10^{-6}	Millionth part of
nano	.000000001	10^{-9}	Billionth part of

These prefixes can be combined with liters and grams.

	Weight	Volume
EXAMPLE:	decigram (dg)	deciliter (dl)
	dekagram (dkg)	dekaliter (dkl)
	hectogram (hg)	hectaliter (hl)
	centigram (cg)	centiliter (cl)
	kilogram (kg)	kiloliter (kl)
	milligram (mg)	milliliter (ml)

NOTE: Some doctors may use the symbol mgm for mg (milligram) and Gm for g (gram). The symbol mcg is the same as μg.

Conversions

REMEMBER: 1 g = 1000 mg

RULES:	1 The metric system is a decimal system. To convert g (large) to mg (small), multiply by 1000 or move the decimal point 3 places to the right (for *1000* times smaller).
	2 To convert mg (small) to g (large), divide by *1000* or move the decimal point 3 places to the left (for *1000* times greater).

EXAMPLE: We know 1000 mg = 1 g.
1500 mg = 1.5 g.
   Divide 1500 mg by 1000 × 1.5 g, or move decimal 3 places
   to the left for converting mg (small) to g (large).
5 g = 5000 mg.
   Multiply 5 g by 1000 = 5000 mg, or move decimal 3 places
   to the right for converting g (large) to mg (small).

Worksheet (Answers on p. 200)

REMEMBER: 1 g = 1000 mg. Move decimals.

1. 1 g = _1000_ mg

2. 2 g = _2000_ mg

3. 1.5 g = _1500_ mg

4. 0.5 g = _500_ mg

5. ½ g = _500_ mg

6. 0.25 g = _250_ mg

7. 0.05 g = _50_ mg

8. 0.1 g = _100_ mg

9. 1.1 g = _1100_ mg

10. 0.3 g = _300_ mg

11. 25 mg = _.025_ g

12. 5 mg = _.005_ g

13. 3000 mg = _3_ g

14. 1500 mg = _1.5_ g

15. 15,000 mg = _15_ g

16. 10 mg = _0.010_ g

17. 100 mg = _0.100_ g

18. 0.5 mg = _0.0005_ g

19. 7.5 mg = _0.0075_ g

20. 20.15 mg = _0.02015_ g

Ratio and proportion

EXAMPLE: 40 mg = _____ g

You already know you can move the decimal point 3 places to the left (divide) and come out with the correct answer. However, now it's time to start setting up a ratio and proportion problem.

1 What we *know* goes on the *left*.
2 What we *want to know* (the x, or unknown) goes on the *right*.

Know	Want to know

1 g:1000 mg::x g:40 mg   PROOF: $1000 \times 0.04 = 40$

$1000x = 40$ $1 \times 40 = 40$

$$\frac{1000x}{1000} = \frac{40}{1000} = 40 \div 1000$$

$$
\begin{array}{r}
.04 \\
1000)\overline{40.00} \\
\underline{40\ 00}
\end{array}
$$

$x = 0.04$ g   Always *label* your answer.

Worksheet   (Answers on p. 200)

Show all work, prove, and label all answers:

REMEMBER: 1 mg = 1000 μg micrograms. mcg
          1 g = 1000 mg
          1 kg (2.2 lb) = 1000 g
          1 L = 1000 ml

Use ratio and proportion:

1. 25 mg = __.025__ g

    .025.

2. 0.064 g = __64__ mg

    .064

3. 4 mg = __.004__ g

    .004,

4. 4.6 g = __4600__ mg

    4.600,

5. 375 ml = __.375__ L

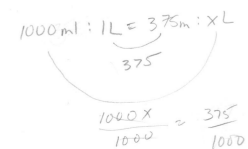

6. 89 kg = _____ g   89,000

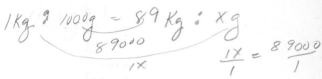

7. 45 mg = _____ μg

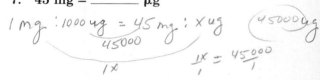

8. 0.6 g = _____ mg   1000.
                                 .6
    1g : 1000mg = 0.6 : x mg   600.0

    1x   ⟨600mg⟩

9. 50 kg = _____ lb

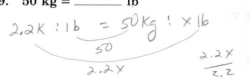

10. 2500 g = _____ lb

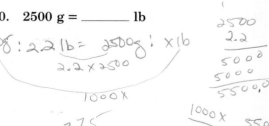

■**51**

Worksheet   (Answers on p. 202)

One-step metric problems

Show all work. Use ratio and proportion, prove and label all work.*

1. Ordered: Valium 5 mg. On hand you have 10 mg tablets. How many tablets will you give?

    $10mg : 1 tab = 5m : x tab.$

    $\dfrac{10x}{10} = \dfrac{5}{10}$ $10\overline{)5.0}$

2. Ordered: 0.1 g of secobarbital. On hand are 0.05 g capsules. How many capsules will you give?

    $.05 gr : 1 tab = 0.1 : x$

    $\dfrac{.05x}{.05}$ $\dfrac{.1}{.05}$ $.05\overline{).10}$

3. Ordered: 500 mg of Achromycin. On hand are 250 mg capsules. How many capsules will you give?

    $250mg : 1 = 500mg = x cap$

    $\dfrac{250x}{250}$ $\dfrac{500}{250}$ $\boxed{2} cap$

4. Ordered: 0.25 g of erythromycin. On hand you have 1 g per 10 ml. How many ml will you give?

    $1g = 10ml = .25g = x ml$

    $\dfrac{1x}{1} = \dfrac{2.50}{1} = 2.50$

5. Ordered: 15 mg of codeine. On hand you have 30 mg tablets. Will you give more or less of what you have on hand? How many tablets will you give?

---

*Only break scored tablets.

Two-step problems

    1000 μg = 1 mg
    1000 mg = 1 g
    1000 g = 1 kg
    1000 ml = 1 L

Two-step ratio and proportion

EXAMPLE: Ordered: 10 mg. On hand you have tablets of 0.002 g each. How many tablets will you give?

Step 1:   Have g on hand. Need to change mg to g because that is what is on hand. What do you know about g and mg?

Know   **Want to know**

1000 mg:1 g::10 mg:x g

*Cancel x out:

$$\frac{\cancel{1000}x}{\cancel{1000}} = \frac{10}{1000} = 10 \div 1000 = 0.01$$

PROOF: 1000 × 0.01 = 10
         1 × 10 = 10

$x = 0.01$ g

The doctor ordered 10 mg. We now know that 10 mg = 0.01 g. Now set up the second step to solve the problem.

Step 2:   **Know**   **Want to know**

0.002 g:1 tab.::0.01 g:x tab.

PROOF: 0.002 × 5 = 0.01
        1 × 0.01 = 0.01

*Cancel x out:

$$\frac{\cancel{0.002}x}{\cancel{0.002}} = \frac{0.01}{0.002} = 0.01 \div 0.002 = 5$$

$x = 5$ tab. of 0.002 g each

---

*There is no need to cancel out if you make sure to put the x on the *left* side and remember to divide the x into the sum on the *right* side of the equation.
†Round answer to nearest tenth of a milliliter.

Worksheet   (Answers on p. 203)

Two-step metric problems. Show all work. Set up ratio and proportion, prove, and label all work. Remember to estimate your answer when you reach the second step.

1. Ordered: 0.75 g of erythromycin. On hand you have 250 mg tablets. How many tablets will you give?

2. Ordered: Valium 10 mg. On hand you have Valium 0.005 g tablets. How many tablets will you give?

3. Ordered: 4 mg of codeine. On hand you have 0.002 g tablets of codeine. How many tablets will you give?

4. Ordered: 75 mg of Demerol IM. On hand you have a vial of 0.050 g per ml. How many ml will you give?*

5. Ordered: chlorpromazine 0.075 g. On hand you have chlorpromazine 25 mg/ml.* How many ml will you give?

*For amounts less than 1 ml, round to the nearest hundredth.
For amounts more than 1 ml, round to the nearest tenth.

6. Ordered: 2 g of Staphcillin. The vial reads: "Add 8.6 ml of diluent to contents of vial. Each ml will contain 500 mg of Staphcillin." How many ml will you administer?

$$1000 \, mg : 1g = x \, mg : 2g$$

$$1x$$

$$\frac{1x}{1} = \frac{2000}{1} \quad 2000$$

$$1 = 2000x$$

$$x = 2000 \, mg$$

$$500 \, mg : 1 \, ml = 2000 \, mg : x \, m$$

$$\frac{2000}{500x} \quad \frac{2000}{500} = \frac{500x}{500}$$

$$= 4m$$

7. Ordered: 500 mg of Gantrisin. Available are Gantrisin 0.25 g tablets. How many tablets will you give? $\left(5g\right)$

$$1000 \, mg : 1g = 500 \, mg : x$$

$$500$$

$$1000x$$

$$\frac{500}{1000} = \frac{1000x}{1000} = \quad \frac{.5}{1000 \overline{)500.0}}$$

$$0.25g : 1tab = .5g : x \, tab$$

$$.5$$

$$.25x$$

$$\frac{.5}{.25} = \frac{.25x}{.25} \quad \frac{2.}{.25 \overline{)50}}$$

$$(2 tab)$$

8. You are to give 0.125 g of Keflin. On hand you have Keflin 50 mg/5 ml. How many ml will you give? The Keflin will be administered in an IV solution.

9. Ordered: Robinul 0.002 g. Available are 1 mg tablets. How many tablets will you give?

10. Ordered: 2 mg of verapamil hydrochloride IV. On hand you have 5 mg/2 ml. How many ml will you give?

Crenshaw, Craig   Rm 145
Age: 83   Dr. Madison
35-409-72-3

MEDICATION ADMINISTRATION RECORD

DATE	DRUG DOSE ROUTE	DATE DC	TIME SCHEDULE	DATE 6/15			DATE			DATE		
				11-7	7-3	3-11	11-7	7-3	3-11	11-7	7-3	3-11
6/15	Valium 5 mg IM IV (PO) R SC		T ID		0900 1300 MS	1700 MS						
	IM IV PO R SC											
	IM IV PO R SC											
	IM IV PO R SC											
	IM IV PO R SC											
	IM IV PO R SC											
	IM IV PO R SC											
	IM IV PO R SC											
	IM IV PO R SC											
	IM IV PO R SC											
	IM IV PO R SC											
	IM IV PO R SC											
	IM IV PO R SC											
	IM IV PO R SC											
	IM IV PO R SC											
	IM IV PO R SC											
	IM IV PO R SC											

PRN/ONE TIME ONLY ORDERS

DATE	DRUG DOSE ROUTE	DATE DC	TIME SCHEDULE	11-7	7-3	3-11	11-7	7-3	3-11	11-7	7-3	3-11
6/15	Codiene 15 mg IM IV (PO) R SC	DC 6/18	q4h prn		1400 MS							
	IM IV PO R SC											
	IM IV PO R SC											
	IM IV PO R SC											
	IM IV PO R SC											
	IM IV PO R SC											
	IM IV PO R SC											
	IM IV PO R SC											

KEY			Signature	Initials	Signature	Initials	Signature	Initials
ABD - ABDOMEN	**LU** - LUQ	**OU** - BOTH EYES	Mary Smith	MS.				
LA - LT. ARM	**O** - NOT GIVEN	**RA** - RT. ARM						
LT - LT. THIGH	**OD** - RT. EYE	**RT** - RT. THIGH						
	OS - LT. EYE	**RU** - RUQ						
IVPB - IV PIGGYBACK	**SQ** - SUBCUTANEOUS							

ALLERGIES
    NKA

■ Metric System Test   (Answers on p. 206)

Use ratio and proportion. Estimate your answer; label and prove answer.

1. 500 mg = ____.5____ g

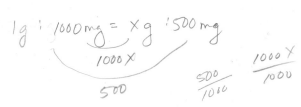
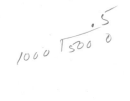
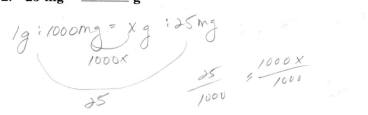
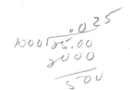

2. 25 mg = ____.025____ g

3. 5 mg = ____5000____ µg

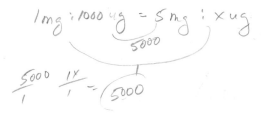

4. 0.2 g = ____200____ mg

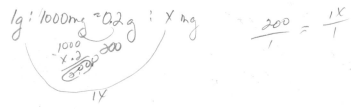
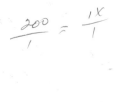

5. 4 g = ____4000____ mg

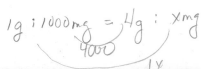

6. Ordered: 10 mg of Valium. On hand you have 0.02 g in each scored tablet. How many tablets will you give? (Is this a one-step or a two-step problem?) Prove.

7. Ordered: 60 mg. On hand you have 20 mg tablets. How many tablets will you give? (Is this a one-step or a two-step problem?)

8. Ordered: 0.75 g. On hand you have 250 mg tablets. How many tablets will you give? (Is this a one-step or two-step problem?)

9. Ordered: 500 mg of Achromycin. On hand are 250 mg tablets. You will give _____ tablets.

10. Digitoxin 0.125 mg tablets are on hand. Give 0.25 mg. How many tablets will you give?

CHAPTER 4

Apothecary/metric system conversions

Objectives
Apothecary

- Memorize symbols for dram, ounce, and drop.
- Calculate one-step apothecary system problems.

Apothecary and metric

- Calculate milligram/grain/gram equivalencies.
- Calculate milliliter/quart/liter/pint and dram/minim/ounce equivalencies.
- Round drops to nearest correct number.
- Calculate metric-apothecary conversion problems.

Apothecary conversions

Explanation

The apothecary system is an imprecise old English system of measurement that is not used very often today. The metric system has virtually replaced the apothecary system. The apothecary system is written in fractions and Roman numerals. This system does not convert exactly to other systems of measurement.

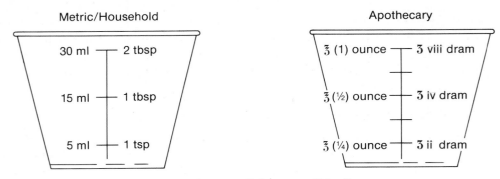

Metric/Household

30 ml — 2 tbsp

15 ml — 1 tbsp

5 ml — 1 tsp

Apothecary

℥ (1) ounce — ℨ viii dram

℥ (½) ounce — ℨ iv dram

℥ (¼) ounce — ℨ ii dram

One ounce medicine cups (30 ml)

■ VOLUME (WET) ■
gtt = drop = minim (♏, ♍, or m) 1 ounce (oz or ℥) = 30 ml = 8 tsp 16 oz (℥) = 1 pint (pt) = 500 ml 2 pt = 1 quart (qt) = 1000 ml 4 qt = 1 gallon (gal) = 4000 ml 32 oz (℥) = 1 qt = 1000 ml

MUST KNOW:
℥ = ounce (oz)
ℨ = dram (dr)
gtt = drop

Equivalents

■ **Table 1.** Approximate equivalents of metric, apothecary, and household measures

Household	Apothecary	Metric
60 drops (gtt)	1 teaspoon (tsp)	5 ml (or cc)*
1 teaspoon (tsp)	1 fluidram (ℨ)	5 ml
1 tablespoon (tbs)	4 fluidrams	15 ml
2 tablespoons (tbs)	8 fluidrams = 1 ounce (℥)	30 ml
1 measuring cup	8 ounces	240 ml
1 pint	16 ounces	500 ml
1 quart	32 ounces	1000 ml

*The abbreviations *ml* and *cc* are used interchangeably; however, *ml* should be used for liquids, *cc* for solids and gases, and *g* for solids.

NOTE: Household measurement conversions may become increasingly important with the trend toward home health care. Also, the apothecary measures and household teaspoons, drams, and tablespoons do not convert accurately to each other or to metric measurements. Apothecary terms of drams and minims are not used today, although they may be seen on syringes and medicine cups.

Roman numerals and Arabic numerals

Roman numerals are used with the apothecary system. Usually Arabic numerals are used for numbers over 9. Fractions are written with Arabic numerals except for $\overline{ss}$ (semis), which stands for one half. If the quantity is composed of a whole number and a fraction, the entire amount is written in Arabic numerals.

Arabic numerals	Capital roman numerals	Small roman numerals
1	I	i
2	II	ii
3	III	iii
4	IV	iv
5	V	v
6	VI	vi
7	VII	vii
8	VIII	viii
9	IX	ix
10	X	x

In the apothecary system the measure or symbol precedes the number. The abbreviation *gr* means grain (originally a grain of wheat).

EXAMPLE: gr xv, gr XV
ℨ i (in handwriting: ℨ i̇)
ʒ ii (in handwriting: ʒ ii̇)
gr $\overline{ss}$ (one half)
gtt ii (drops)

NOTE: Don't confuse ℨ (dram) and ʒ (ounce).

Ratio and proportion

EXAMPLE: You have a vial of caffeine containing gr 1½ per ml. Ordered: caffeine gr 3¾. How many ml will you give?

What was ordered and what you *have* on hand are in the same system; therefore, it is a one-step problem.

REMEMBER: *Have* or *know* goes on the *left*.

Have   Want to know

gr 1½:1 ml::gr 3¾:x ml   PROOF: $1 \times 3¾ = 3¾$

$$\frac{1½x}{1½} = \frac{3¾}{1½} = \frac{15}{4} \div \frac{3}{2} = \frac{15}{4} \times \frac{2}{3} = \frac{30}{12} = 2½$$

$1½ \times 2½ = 3¾$

$x = 2½$ ml $= 2.5$ ml

4A Worksheet   (Answers on p. 206)

Using ratio and proportion, prove:

1. You are to give codeine gr i. You have codeine gr $\overline{ss}$ per ml. How many ml will you give?

2. You are to give ASA gr XV. You have ASA gr V per tablet. How many tablets will you give?

3. Ordered: morphine sulfate gr ⅙. You have on hand a vial containing morphine sulfate gr ⅛ per ml. How many ml will you give? (For amounts over 1 ml, calculate to tenths; for amounts under 1 ml, calculate to hundredths.)

4. On hand you have a can of Metamucil containing ʒ viii. You are to give Metamucil ʒ ii. How many teaspoons will you mix with juice or water? How many ml is this?

5. You are to give ℥ s̄s̄ of Maalox. On hand you have a bottle containing Maalox ℥ viii. How many ml will you give?

6. You are to give codeine sulfate gr ⅙ SC. On hand you have codeine sulfate gr ¼ per ml. How many ml will you give? Your immediate reaction will be to give _____ (more or less) than 1 ml. (Calculate to hundredths. Do not round.)

7. You are to give Nembutal gr īs̄s̄. On hand you have Nembutal gr s̄s̄. How many capsules will you give?

8. Ordered: atropine gr ¹⁄₂₀₀. On hand you have an ampule of atropine labeled gr ¹⁄₁₅₀ per 0.5 ml. How many ml will you give?

9. On hand you have Gantrisin tablets gr V. Doctor ordered Gantrisin tablets gr 15. How many tablets will you give?

10. Ordered: ℥ s̄s̄ of cough syrup. How many ml will you give?

Apothecary and metric conversions

Equivalency tables

■ VOLUME ■
1000 milliliters (ml) = 1 liter (L) = 1 quart (qt)
1 ml = 1 cubic centimeter (cc)
500 ml = 1 pint (pt)
30 ml = 1 ounce (℥) or 8 drams (ℨ)
5 ml = 1 dram = 1 tsp = 4 or 5 ml
1 ml = 15 or 16 minims (♏)
1 m̅ = 1 drop (gtt)

■ WEIGHT ■
1000 mg = 1 gram (g) = gr XV (15)
500 mg = 0.5 g = gr Viiss
60–67* mg = gr ĭi
0.6 mg = gr 1/100
0.4 mg = gr 1/150
0.3 mg = gr 1/200
0.2 mg = gr 1/300

*The value 60 mg is more commonly used (see diagram below). The value gr 1/60 = 1 mg is more commonly used than gr 1/67.

Apothecary system does not convert exactly to metric.

A GOOD WAY TO REMEMBER:

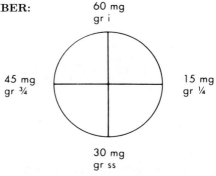

"The Metric Clock"

EXAMPLE: 0.1 g is different from 1.0 g.

RULE:	Apothecary is made definitive by adding a dot for clarification of the number one. The symbol precedes the number. Roman numerals are frequently used.

EXAMPLE: gr i (1) or gr vii$\overline{\text{ss}}$ (7½)

EXAMPLE: gr xv

When proving answers from apothecary to metric, you will notice a slight difference (one tenth) because the apothecary system is not so accurate as the metric system. Proving answers *must* be done with the original answer and then rounded off if necessary.

EXAMPLE:

Know   **Want to know**

1.0 g:gr $15::x$ g:gr 5

$15x = 5$

$x = 0.333$ g

PROOF: $1.0 \times 5 = 5$

$15 \times 0.33 = 4.95 = 5$

RULE:	When working with the metric system, note that the symbol *follows* the Arabic number.

EXAMPLE: 0.5 g

Rounding Off

RULE:	Drops are so small that it is impossible to divide them into parts. Therefore any remainder of 0.5 or above is given the next highest number.

EXAMPLE: Drops   6.7 gtt   Give 7 gtt.

Syringes are calibrated in tenths as well as whole numbers or ml. Therefore if the answer is 1.7 ml, do NOT round off to 2 ml.

RULE:	Tenths and hundredths can be measured accurately on syringes.

EXAMPLE: 1.57 ml   Give 1.6 ml in a 2 or 3 ml syringe.

The 7 in 1.57 is greater than 5, so the next highest number can be added to the 5, making the correct dosage 1.6 ml.

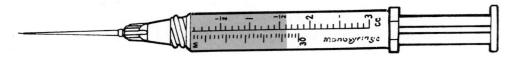

EXAMPLE: 0.73 ml   Give 0.73 ml.

Use a TB syringe for amounts less than 1 ml when a very precise dosage is indicated.

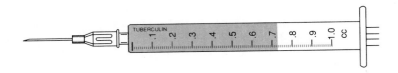

4B Worksheet   (Answers on p. 209)

MEMORIZE: 1 g = gr 15
                60 mg = gr i

One-step problems

Use ratio and proportion, prove answers, and label answers:

1. gr 10 = _.66_ g

$1g : gr\ 15 = x\ g : gr\ 10$
$\frac{15x}{15} \quad \frac{10}{15} = \frac{15x}{15}$

$15)\overline{\begin{array}{r}.66\\10.00\\90\\100\end{array}}$

4. gr ¾ = _____ mg

2. 0.5 g = gr _7.5_

$1g : gr\ 15 = 0.5 : x\ gr$
$\frac{}{1x}$

$15 \begin{array}{r} 2 \\ .5 \\ 7.5 \end{array}$

5. gr ¹⁄₁₅₀ = _____ mg

3. gr viiss = _.5_ g
     7½

■ 66

Worksheet   (Answers on p. 210)

Figure these in your head. Complete the following equivalents:

1. 1 mg = _.001_ g

2. 5 g = _5000_ mg

3. 1 g = gr _15_

4. gr 7½ = _.05_ g

5. 15 mg = gr _gr ¼_

6. 1 L = _1000_ ml

7. 30 ml = _1 oz_ ʒ

8. 1 ml = _15·16_ gtt

9. 2 ʒ = _8 ml_ ml

10. 1 cc = _1_ ml

11. 1 kg = _1000_ g

12. gr ¹⁄₂₀₀ = _0.3_ mg

13. gr iii = _180_ mg

14. ʒ i = _30_ ml

15. 1 tsp = _5_ ml

16. 1 gtt = _60_ ℳ

17. Which is smaller: mg or gr? _mg_   gr i = 60 mg

18. Which is larger: g or gr? _g_

19. Which is larger: 30 ml or ½ oz? _30 m_

20. Which is larger: 15 ml or ʒi? _15 ml_

Worksheet   (Answers on p. 210)

MUST KNOW:

1 g = gr 15
gr i = 60 mg
ʒ i = 30 ml
ʒ i = 5 ml

1. You are to give Milk of Magnesia (MOM) ʒ iss. How many ml will you give?

   1½

   1 g = 30 ml   = 45 ml

2. Ordered: atropine sulfate gr ¹⁄₃₀₀ to be given on call to the O.R. On hand you have 0.50 mg per 0.5 ml. How many ml will you give?

   60/300 = ⅕ = 0.2 mg/5+1000

   60 ¹⁄₃₀₀ / 1   60mg : gr i = x mg : gr ¹⁄₃₀₀   ⅓ = ¹ˣ/₁ =   X = .2mg

3. You need to give Robitussin ℥ ii p.o. How many ml will you give?

2 droms = 2 tsp

10 ml

4. Ordered: Demerol gr ¾. On hand you have a vial of Demerol labeled 75 mg/cc. How many ml will you give?

75 mg/cc   gr 3/4

$75 mg : 1 ml = 45 mg : X ml$
$\overline{45}$

$60 mg : gr 1 = mg x : gr 3/4$ or $.75$

$45 mg = \dfrac{75 x}{0.6 ml}$

5. You are to give ASA (acetylsalicylic acid) 0.6 g. The tablets on hand are labeled ASA gr v. How many tablets will you give?

gr V : 1 tab   0.6 g

6. Ordered: 650 mg ASA for a temperature above 101° F. Your patient developed a fever of 102° F. How many tablets of ASA gr 5 per tablet will you give?

7. You are to give caffeine sodium benzoate gr viiss. You have an ampule labeled caffeine sodium benzoate 0.5 g in 2.0 cc. How many ml will you give?

8. You have a 2-ml ampule of caffeine Na benzoate containing gr viiss. If the physician orders gr V, how many ml will you give?

$gr 7½ : 2 ml = gr V : X ml$

10

$\dfrac{10}{7.5} = 1.3 m$

7.½ X

9. Ordered: Nembutal 100 mg. On hand you have Nembutal gr $\overline{\text{iss}}$. How many capsules will you give?

10. You have an ampule of Amytal Sodium gr ii/1.25 ml. Doctor ordered 30 mg IV. How many ml will you give?

4E **Worksheet** (Answers on p. 212)

1. Ordered: gr ¹⁄₂₀₀ scopolamine SC injection. On hand is a vial of scopolamine that reads 1 ml = gr ¹⁄₁₅₀. How many ml would you give?

2. In the narcotic box the morphine is labeled M.S. gr ¼ per 1 cc. Ordered is M.S. gr ⅙. How many ml would you give (to nearest tenth)?
   Before you begin this problem, will give more or less than 1 ml?

3. Ordered: codeine gr ½ p.o. On hand are 15-mg tablets. How many tablets would you give?

4. Penicillin 300,000 U IM is ordered every 4 hours. On hand is a 10-ml vial of penicillin labeled 400,000 U per 1 ml. How many minims would you give for 1 dose?

5. Gantrisin 0.50 g (oral) is ordered. On hand is Gantrisin 250 mg per tablet. How many tablets would you give?

6. Demerol 75 mg IM is ordered stat. On hand is Demerol 100 mg per 2 ml. How many ml would you give (nearest tenth)?

7. Atropine gr $\frac{1}{300}$ by injection is ordered for a patient going to surgery. The nurse has a bottle from stock labeled scopolamine gr $\frac{1}{150}$ ml. How many ml of scopolamine would you give?

8. Chloral hydrate gr viiss̄ is ordered for sleep. On hand is a bottle marked chloral hydrate. One tablet is 0.25 g. How many tablets would you give?

9. MOM with cascara ʒ s̄s̄ is ordered. How many ml will you give?

10. Morphine gr $\frac{1}{200}$ IM is ordered. On hand you have an ampule labeled morphine 0.4 mg per ml. How many ml will you give?

Lester, Rhona   Rm 590
Age: 25   Dr. Salts
62-109-83-7

MEDICATION ADMINISTRATION RECORD

DATE	DRUG	DOSE	ROUTE	DATE DC	TIME SCHEDULE	DATE 7/1			DATE			DATE		
						11-7	7-3	3-11	11-7	7-3	3-11	11-7	7-3	3-11
7/1	ASA	gr 5	IM IV (PO) R SC		QD		0230 JM							
			IM IV PO R SC											
			IM IV PO R SC											
			IM IV PO R SC											
			IM IV PO R SC											
			IM IV PO R SC											
			IM IV PO R SC											
			IM IV PO R SC											
			IM IV PO R SC											
			IM IV PO R SC											
			IM IV PO R SC											
			IM IV PO R SC											
			IM IV PO R SC											
			IM IV PO R SC											
			IM IV PO R SC											
			IM IV PO R SC											
			IM IV PO R SC											
			IM IV PO R SC											

PRN/ONE TIME ONLY ORDERS

DATE	DRUG	DOSE	ROUTE	DATE DC	TIME SCHEDULE	11-7	7-3	3-11	11-7	7-3	3-11	11-7	7-3	3-11
7/3	Morphine 15 mg		(IM) IV PO R SC		q3h prn		1800 LT JM							
			IM IV PO R SC											
			IM IV PO R SC											
			IM IV PO R SC											
			IM IV PO R SC											
			IM IV PO R SC											
			IM IV PO R SC											

KEY				Signature	Initials	Signature	Initials	Signature	Initials
ABD - ABDOMEN	**O** - NOT GIVEN	**RA** - RT. ARM		Jane Mack	JM				
LA - LT. ARM	**OD** - RT. EYE	**RT** - RT. THIGH							
LT - LT. THIGH	**OS** - LT. EYE	**RU** - RUQ							
IVPB - iV PIGGYBACK	**SQ** - SUBCUTANEOUS								

LU - LUQ

OU - BOTH EYES

ALLERGIES
  NKDA

■ 71

■ Apothecary/Metric System Test   (Answers on p. 214)

Use ratio and proportion; prove and label your answers.

1. Ordered is Pantopon gr ⅙ IM q.4h. p.r.n. The vial on hand is labeled Pantopon gr ¼ in 1 ml. How much will you give?

2. You are to give morphine sulfate gr ⅙. The morphine available is labeled gr ½ in 1 ml. How many ml will you give?

3. Ordered: elixir of terpin hydrate (ETH) with codeine ℥ iii. This is equal to how many ml?

4. You are to give atropine gr ¹⁄₂₀₀. On hand is a Tubex cartridge with gr ¹⁄₁₅₀ in 0.5 ml. How many ml will you give?

5. You have a vial of caffeine containing gr 1½ per ml. You are to give gr ¾. How many ml will you give?

6. Ordered: ASA (acetylsalicylic acid) 300 mg. On hand is aspirin labeled gr V per tablet. How many tablets will you give?

7. gr 10 = _____ g

9. gr viiss = _____ mg

8. gr xxx = _____ mg

10. gr ¾ = _____ mg

CHAPTER 5

Medications from powder and crystals

Objectives

- Reconstitute medications from powders and crystals.
- Determine the best dilution strength to mix for the ordered amount of medication.

Explanation

Diluting powder or crystals in vials

Directions for dissolving drugs in vials can be found in the accompanying literature. Information given will be the volume of the powder after it is dissolved in NS or distilled water. For instance, the directions may read: "Add 1.4 ml NS to make 2 ml of reconstituted solution." These directions tell the user that the powder takes up to 0.6 ml of space.

$$1.4 \text{ ml} + 0.6 \text{ ml} = 2 \text{ ml}$$

RULE:	Read the label to find out how many units, grams, milligrams, or micrograms are in each ml of the reconstituted drug.

EXAMPLE: DIRECTIONS: Add 1.4 ml distilled water (sterile) to make 600,000 U of penicillin per 2 ml.

Ordered: 300,000 U penicillin IM q6h.

Have   Want

2 ml:600,000 U::x ml:300,000 U   PROOF:

$6x = 6$ $2 \times 3 = 6$

$x = 1$ ml $6 \times 1 = 6$

Give 1 ml of reconstituted solution for each 300,000 U.
Shade in syringe to show 1 ml.

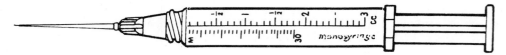

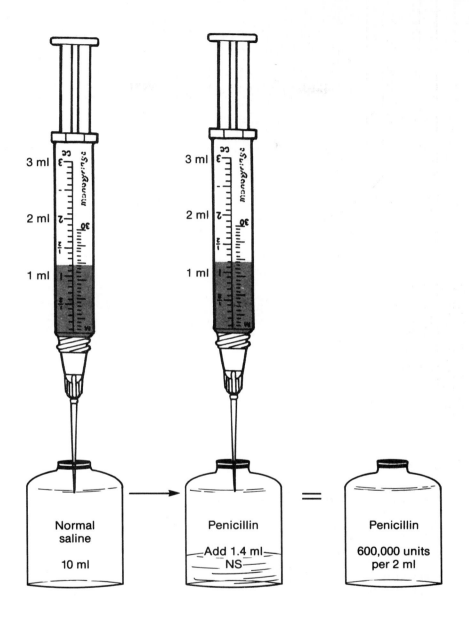

Normal
saline

10 ml

Penicillin

Add 1.4 ml
NS

Penicillin

600,000 units
per 2 ml

Many solutions are unstable after being reconstituted. Read labels carefully for directions on storing them in the refrigerator or in a dark place. There is usually a time limit or expiration date on the vial. It is important to date, label, and initial all reconstituted medications.

Worksheet (Answers on p. 215)

1. Ordered: Kefzol (cefazolin sodium) 300 mg IM.
   - How many ml of diluent will be used?
   - How many mg/ml will it make?
   - What is the shelf life of the medication after reconstitution?
   - How many ml will you give? Shade in syringe.

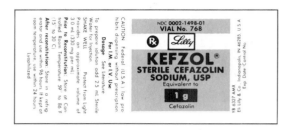

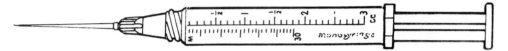

2. Ordered: Prostaphlin 450 mg IM.
   - How many ml of sterile water for injection will be used?
   - How many mg/ml will it make?
   - What is the shelf life of the medication after reconstitution?
   - How many ml will you give? Shade in syringe.

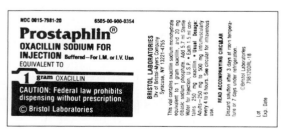

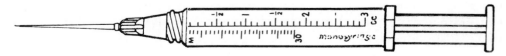

3. Ordered: 500 mg Polycillin-N IM q6h.
   - How many ml of diluent are needed to reconstitute?
   - How many mg/ml will it make?
   - What is the shelf life of the medication?
   - How many ml will you give? Shade in syringe.

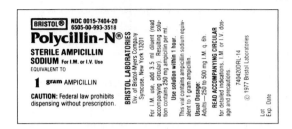

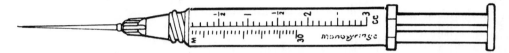

4. Ordered: 300 mg Prostaphlin IM q4h.
   - How many ml of diluent should be used to reconstitute?
   - How many mg/ml will it make?
   - What is the shelf life of the medication?
   - How many ml will you give? Shade in syringe.

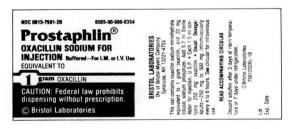

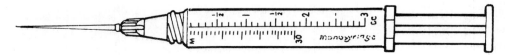

5. Ordered: 1000 mg Staphcillin IM q6h.
   - How many ml of diluent should be used to reconstitute?
   - How many g/ml will it make?
   - What is the shelf life of the medication?
   - How many ml of medication will you give? Shade in syringe.

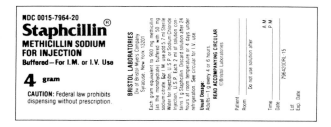

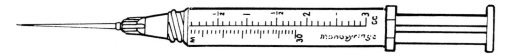

6. Ordered: Penicillin G Potassium 750,000 U IM.
   - Which strength will you use?
   - How many ml of diluent will be used?
   - What is the shelf life of the medication after reconstitution?
   - How many ml of medication will you give? Shade in syringe.

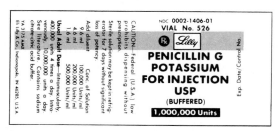

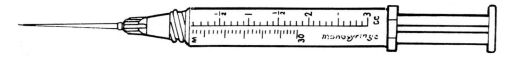

7. Ordered: 750 mg Ticar IM.
   - How many ml of diluent will be added?
   - How many g/ml will it make?
   - What is the shelf life of the medication?
   - How many ml will you give? Shade in syringe.

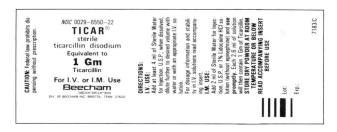

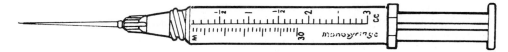

Worksheet   (Answers on p. 217)

1. Ordered: Prostaphlin (sodium oxacillin) 500 mg IM. You have a multidose vial that reads: "Prostaphlin; add 5.7 ml sterile water for injection." Each 1.5 ml of solution contains 0.25 g. How many ml will you give? Shade in syringe.

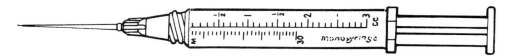

2. Ordered: potassium penicillin G (Pfizerpen) 300,000 U IM. You have a multidose vial containing 1 million U and the following directions:

Ml of diluent added	Units per ml
19.6	50,000
9.6	100,000
3.6	250,000
1.6	500,000

Which dilution will you make and label? What amount will you give? Shade in syringe.

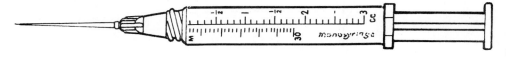

3. Ordered: 200 mg Keflin IM q4h. Available is Keflin (cephalothin sodium) 1 g in a 10 ml vial. Each g of Keflin should be diluted with 4 ml of sterile water for injection. The reconstituted material will provide two 500-mg doses of 2.2 ml each. How many ml will you give? Shade in syringe.

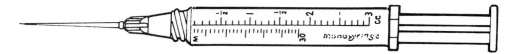

4. Ordered: 125 mg Kefzol (cefazolin sodium) IM. Available is cefazolin sodium 500 mg with the following directions for reconstitution: "Add 2 ml sterile water for injection or 0.9% sodium chloride for injection. Provides approximate volume of 2.2 ml (225 mg/ml) after reconstitution. Store in refrigerator. Protect from light, and use within 96 hours. If kept at room temperature, use within 24 hours." How many ml will you give? Shade in syringe.

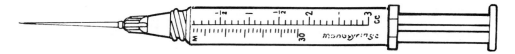

5. Ordered: Totacillin-N (sodium ampicillin) 500 mg IM stat. Available is a powdered form labeled "0.50 g for IV or IM use. For IM use, add at least 1.7 ml sterile water for injection, USP. Use solution within 1 hour after reconstituting." Each ml will contain 0.25 g. How many ml will you give? Shade in syringe.

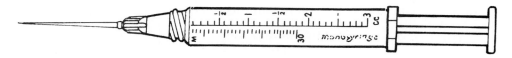

6. Ordered: Achromycin 500 mg IV volutrol stat. Available is Achromycin (tetracycline hydrochloride) 0.50 g per 2.5 ml. How many ml will you prepare?

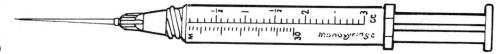

7. Ordered: Kantrex (kanamycin sulfate) 300 mg IM. Directions on bottle read: "Add 2.7 ml sterile water for injection to make 1 g per 3 ml." After reconstitution, how many ml will you give? Shade in syringe.

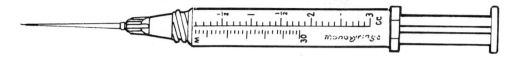

8. Ordered: 1.2 million units of penicillin. You have a 10 ml vial containing 0.5 million U/ml. How many ml will you give? How many ml will be left in the vial? How many units of penicillin will be left in the vial? How many ml will you give? Shade in syringe.

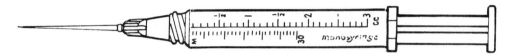

9. A vial of penicillin contains 5 million U. Doctor ordered 500,000 U. You wish to make each ml equal 500,000 U. Approximately how many ml of diluent will you use?

10. A vial is labeled 500,000 U/ml. Doctor ordered 800,000 U IM q4h. How many ml will you give? Shade in syringe.

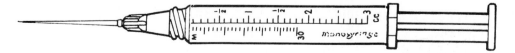

Vox, Harry   Rm 401C
Age: 62   Dr. Baines
31-604-36-2

MEDICATION ADMINISTRATION RECORD

DATE	DRUG	DOSE	ROUTE	DATE DC	TIME SCHEDULE	DATE 8/25			DATE			DATE		
						11-7	7-3	3-11	11-7	7-3	3-11	11-7	7-3	3-11
8/25	Keflol 300 mg		(IM) IV PO R SC		BID	0700 7B LU	1900 7B LU							
			IM IV PO R SC											
			IM IV PO R SC											
			IM IV PO R SC											
			IM IV PO R SC		·									
			IM IV PO R SC											
			IM IV PO R SC											
			IM IV PO R SC											
			IM IV PO R SC											
			IM IV PO R SC											
			IM IV PO R SC											
			IM IV PO R SC											
			IM IV PO R SC											
			IM IV PO R SC											
			IM IV PO R SC											
			IM IV PO R SC											
			IM IV PO R SC											

PRN/ONE TIME ONLY ORDERS

			IM IV PO R SC											
			IM IV PO R SC											
			IM IV PO R SC											
			IM IV PO R SC											
			IM IV PO R SC											
			IM IV PO R SC											
			IM IV PO R SC											
			IM IV PO R SC											

Signature	Initials	Signature	Initials	Signature	Initials
Fay Baye	7B				

KEY

	LU - LUQ	**OU** - BOTH EYES			
ABD - ABDOMEN	**O** - NOT GIVEN	**RA** - RT. ARM			
LA - LT. ARM	**OD** - RT. EYE	**RT** - RT. THIGH			
LT - LT. THIGH	**OS** - LT. EYE	**RU** - RUQ			

IVPB - IV PIGGYBACK   **SQ** - SUBCUTANEOUS

ALLERGIES

aspirin

■ Medications From Powder and Crystals Test (Answers on p. 219) Use ratio and proportion.

1. Ordered: penicillin G 300,000 U IM q4h. Pharmacy sent a vial with 3 million U penicillin G in dry crystal form. Directions were to dilute with 4.2 ml NS to make 5 ml. After dilution, the vial contains 3 million units per 5 ml U. How many ml will you give?

2. Ordered: Keflin 0.5 g IM q6h. Pharmacy sent a vial of sodium cephalothin (Keflin) 1 g in powder form. Directions read: "Add 4 ml sterile water to make two 0.5 g doses of 2.2 ml each." How many ml will you give?

3. Dilute a vial containing 100,000 U of Polycillin (ampicillin) so that each ml contains 50,000 U. Approximately how much distilled water will you need to add to the vial to get 50,000 U/ml? Shade in syringe.

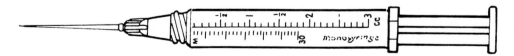

4. A vial contains 500,000 units of carbenicillin. Prepare the dry powder to contain a solution of 250,000 U/ml. Approximately how much distilled water will you need to add to the vial? Shade in syringe.

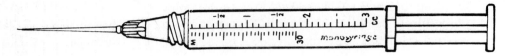

5. Ordered: 400,000 U Keflin. You have a vial with 600,000 U/ml. How many ml will you give? Shade in syringe.

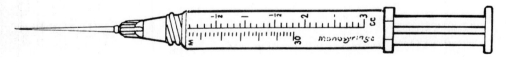

CHAPTER 6

Basic intravenous calculations

Objectives

- Memorize two-step formula for calculating IV flow rates.
- Given an order for IV solutions, calculate milliliters per hour.
- Given the drop factor, calculate drops per minute.
- Use drop factor for microdrip tubing.
- Determine whether to start at step 1 or step 2 of IV rate calculation.
- Calculate IV flow rates.
- Calculate infusion time.

Explanation

There are two steps in IV calculations. The first step is to find out how many *ml per hour* the IV must infuse. The second step is to calculate the *drops per minute* needed to infuse the ml/hr.

Analyze your problem. If the doctor ordered the IV to infuse for 8 hours, you must begin at step 1 to figure the ml/hr. If the order *reads* the IV is to infuse at 75 ml/hr, start at step 2.

RULE: When the total volume is given, calculate the ml/hr.

Step 1: $\dfrac{\text{Total volume (TV)}}{\text{Total time (TT)}} = \text{ml/hr}$

EXAMPLE: ORDERED: 2000 ml D5W (dextrose 5% in water) to be infused in 8 hours. The problem is to find out how many ml/hr the patient must receive for the 2000 ml to be infused in 8 hours.

Formula:

$$\frac{\text{Total volume (TV)}}{\text{Total time (TT)}} = \text{ml/hr}$$

$$\frac{\text{Total volume (TV)}}{\text{Total time (TT)}} = \frac{2000 \text{ ml}}{8 \text{ hr}} = \text{ml/hr}$$

$$\frac{\text{TV}}{\text{TT}} = \frac{2000}{8} = 2000 \div 8 = 250 \text{ ml/hr}$$

We now know that to get 2000 ml of fluid in 8 hours the patient must get 250 ml/hr. Now calculate how many drops are needed per *minute* to infuse 250 ml/hr.

Explanation

The drop factor is the number of drops in 1 ml (or 1 cc). The diameter of the tube where the drop enters the drip chamber varies from one manufacturer to another. The bigger the tube, the fatter the drop (Fig. 1, *A*); thus it may take only 10 gtt to make a ml. The smallest unit is the microdrop (60 gtt/ml) (Fig. 1, *B*). This is used for people who can tolerate only small amounts of fluid. Drop factors of 10, 15, and 60 (microdrip) are the most common. The drop factor is found on the IV tubing box.

RULE:	When the ml/hr is given, calculate the gtt/min.

Step 2: $\dfrac{\text{Drop factor or gtt/ml (IV box)}}{\text{Time in minutes}} \times \text{Total hourly volume (V/hr)} = \text{gtt/min}$

EXAMPLE: ORDERED: D5W to infuse at 250 ml/hr. Drop factor is 10.

$$\frac{\text{Drop factor (Df)}}{\text{Time (min)}} \times \text{V/hr} \qquad \frac{10 \text{ (Df)}}{60 \text{ (min)}} \times 250 \text{ (V/hr)}$$

$$\frac{10}{60} \times \frac{250}{1} = \frac{1}{6} \times \frac{250}{1} = \frac{250}{6} = 41.6 \text{ or } 42 \text{ drops/min}$$

EXAMPLE: ORDERED: Antibiotic to infuse at 100 ml in 30 minutes. Drop factor is 15.

$$\frac{\text{Df}}{\text{Time (min)}} \times \text{V/hr} \qquad \frac{15 \text{ (Df)}}{30 \text{ (min)}} \times 100 \text{ (V/hr)}$$

$$\frac{15}{30} \times \frac{100}{1} = \frac{1}{2} \times \frac{100}{1} = \frac{100}{2} = 50 \text{ drops/min}$$

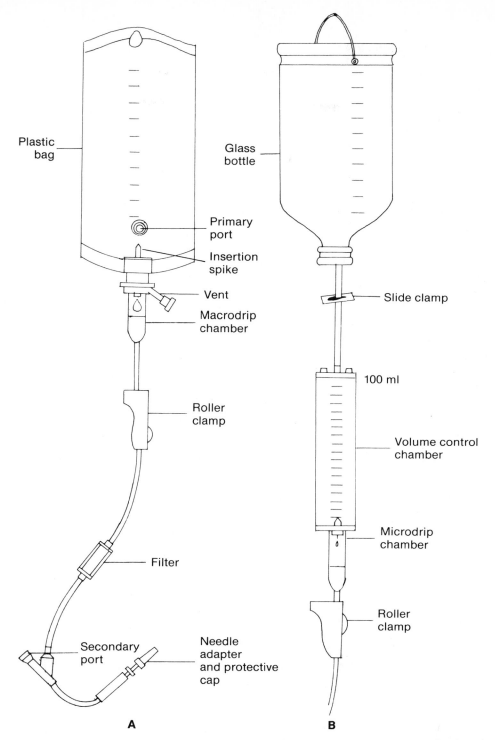

Fig. 1. Intravenous administration sets. **A,** With macrodrip chamber. **B,** With microdrip chamber. Microdrip volume chamber can deliver 100 ml/hr. (From Clayton BD and Stock YN: Basic pharmacology for nurses, ed 9, St Louis, 1989, Mosby–Year Book.)

SUMMARY: Two-step IV flow rate calculations

Step 1: $\dfrac{TV}{TT}$ = ml/hr

Step 2: $\dfrac{Df}{Min} \times$ V/hr = gtt/min   Remember to reduce fraction *before* multiplying.

or

$\dfrac{D}{M} \times$ V = gtt/min   DMV (Department of Motor Vehicles) may be easier to remember.

REMEMBER: Reduce the fraction $\dfrac{Df}{Min}$ or $\dfrac{D}{M}$ *before* multiplying by the volume.

Which would you rather calculate?

$\dfrac{12}{60} \times 60$ or $\dfrac{1}{5} \times 60$

The reduced fraction is easier to calculate.

■ ABBREVIATIONS FOR COMMON INTRAVENOUS SOLUTIONS ■	
NS	Normal saline 0.9%
1/2 NS	Normal saline 0.45%
D/RL	Dextrose with Ringer's lactate solution
D5W or 5% D/W	Dextrose 5% in water
RL or RLS	Ringer's lactate solution (electrolytes)
Isolytes	Electrolyte solutions
D5NS	Dextrose 5% in normal saline

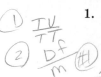

6A Worksheet* (Answers on p. 220)

1. Ordered: 1000 ml to be infused in 8 hours. How many gtt/min if the drop factor is 10?
   Start at step ___1___.

$$\frac{1000ml}{8hrs} = 8\overline{)1000} \quad \frac{125 ml}{8}$$

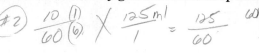

2. Ordered: 200 ml to be infused in an hour. If drop factor is 12, how many gtt/min?
   Start at step ___2___.

$$\frac{Drops}{mn} \frac{12 (1)}{60 (6)} \quad \frac{200 ml}{1} (Volume) = \frac{200 ml}{5} \quad 5\overline{)2000}$$

$$\frac{40 gtts}{mn}$$

3. Ordered: 100 ml to be infused in 30 minutes. How many gtt/min if drop factor is 10?
   Start at step ___2___.

$$\frac{10(1)}{30(3)} \times \frac{100 ml}{1} = \frac{100 ml}{3} = 3\overline{)100} \quad 33.3 \quad 10.0 \qquad 33 gtts/mn$$

4. Ordered: 1500 ml to be infused in 12 hours. If drop factor is 15, how many gtt/min?
   Start at step ___1___.

$$\frac{1500}{12} = 12\overline{)1500} \quad 125/1$$

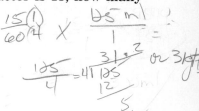

5. Ordered: 50 ml to be infused in an hour. How many gtt/min with micro-drip?

---

*FORMULA: $\frac{TV}{TT}$ = ml/hr $\frac{D}{M}$ × V/hr = gtt/min

To count gtt/min: Count the drops in 6 seconds and multiply by 10.

6. Ordered: 1500 ml to be infused in 8 hours. How many ml/hr?
   a. How many gtt/min with drop factor of 10?

   b. How many gtt/min with drop factor of 15?

7. Ordered: 75 ml to be infused in 45 minutes. Drop factor is 10. How many gtt/min?

8. Ordered: 250 ml to be infused in 90 minutes. Drop factor is microdrip. How many gtt/min?

9. Ordered: 150 ml to infuse in 40 minutes. Drop factor is 15 gtt/ml. How many gtt/min?

10. Ordered: 1000 ml to infuse at 150 ml/hr. Drop factor is 20. How many gtt/min?

Worksheet (Answers on p. 221)

1. You have 2000 ml 5% D/W being infused for 24 hours. How many ml/hr?

2. You have 1500 ml NS. Drop factor is 15. Solution is to be given for an 8-hour period. How many ml/hr? How many gtt/min?

3. Solution of 3000 ml D5W is being infused for 24 hours with 1.5 g carbenicillin. Drop factor is 60 (microdrip). How many gtt/min? With which step will you begin?

4. You have 500 ml 0.45% NS infusing for 4 hours. Drop factor is 15. How many gtt/min?

5. Doctor ordered 1000 ml to be infused for 12 hours on microdrip. How many gtt/min will you regulate the flow?

6. Order calls for 100 ml gentamicin to be infused within 30 minutes. Drop factor is 12. How many gtt/min?

7. Ordered: 2000 ml for 24 hours. Drop factor is 15. How many gtt/min?

8. Ordered: 250 ml D5W is to be infused for 10 hours on a microdrip. How many gtt/min?

9. Ordered: 1500 ml of Ringer's lactate solution to run for 12 hours. How many ml/hr? Drop factor is 15. How many gtt/min?

10. Write your two-step formula again.

    Step 1

    Step 2

Worksheet   (Answers on p. 223)

1. Ordered: 100 ml/hr. How many gtt/min if drop factor is 10? (Start at step 1 or step 2?)

2. Ordered: 1000 ml to be infused in 6 hours. How many gtt/min if drop factor is 15? (Start at step 1 or step 2?)

3. Ordered: 50 ml to be infused in 30 minutes. How many gtt/min if drop factor is 10? (Start at step 1 or step 2?)

4. Ordered: 100 ml to be infused in 60 minutes. How many gtt/min if a microdrip is used? (Start at step 1 or step 2?)

5. Ordered: 2000 ml to be infused in 12 hours. Drop factor is 60.
    a. How many ml/hr?
    b. How many gtt/min?

6. Ordered: 100 ml to be infused in 30 minutes. Drop factor is 12. How many gtt/min?

7. Ordered: 1500 ml 0.45% NS in 24 hours. Drop factor is 10. How many gtt/min?

8. Ordered: 500 ml in 8 hours by microdrip. How many gtt/min?

9. Ordered: 1000 ml Ringer's lactate solution at 75 ml/hr. Drop factor is 15. How many gtt/min?

10. Ordered: D5W continuous infusion at 85 ml/hr. Drop factor is 20. How many gtt/min?

Explanation

IVPB is an acronym for intravenous piggyback (Fig. 2). When special medications are ordered intermittently, the primary IV can be bypassed by introducing the medication through a special entry or portal. Piggyback (PB) medications are infused intermittently via the existing IV line. An extension tubing with a needle attachment is inserted into the portal or entry site. The PB infusion is usually 50 to 250 ml of medicated solution.

Elevating the IVPB 12 inches above the existing IV allows the PB to infuse by gravity. When the PB is finished, the *existing* IV will resume at the rate set for the IVPB. The nurse must remember to regulate the IV to the *previous* rate.

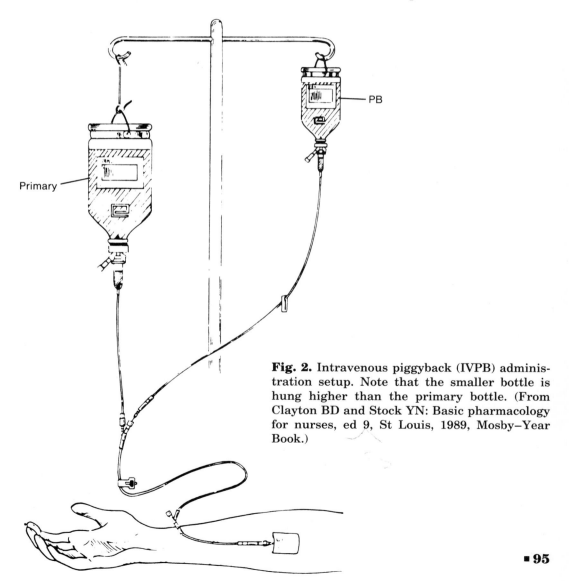

Fig. 2. Intravenous piggyback (IVPB) administration setup. Note that the smaller bottle is hung higher than the primary bottle. (From Clayton BD and Stock YN: Basic pharmacology for nurses, ed 9, St Louis, 1989, Mosby–Year Book.)

RULE:	Return the primary IV to the original rate after the PB has been infused.

Volutrol and buritrol administer controlled amounts of medication solution. The IV tubing has a special pouch or container that holds 100 ml. Medication is injected into the volutrol/buritrol via the portal. The bag or container is then filled with the primary IV solution and the primary IV clamped until the medication has been infused. The medication can be controlled (gtt/min) by the regulator below the volutrol/buritrol.

6D **Worksheet**   (Answers on p. 224)

1. Ordered: Keflin 4 g in 100 ml IVPB to be infused over 1 hour. The drop factor is 15.
   - How many gtt/min?

2. Ordered: ampicillin 500 mg in 50 ml IVPB to be infused in 20 minutes.
   - How many gtt/min if drop factor is 15?

3. Ordered: gentamicin 80 mg in 50 ml IVPB to be infused in 30 minutes.
   - How many gtt/min if drop factor is 60?

4. Ordered: Aq. penicillin 600,000 U in 100 ml IVPB to be infused in 1 hour. The drop factor is 12.
   - How many gtt/min?

5. Ordered: 250 ml NS to be infused at 60 gtt/min. The drop factor is 20 gtt/ml.
   - How long will it take to infuse?

6. Ordered: 2000 ml D5W to be infused at 40 gtt/min. The drop factor is 15 gtt/ml.
   - How long will it take to infuse?

7. Ordered: Kantrex 300 mg in 150 ml IVPB. Label reads to infuse in 40 to 60 minutes. Drop factor is microdrip.
   - How many gtt/min to infuse in 40 minutes?
   - What is the slowest infusion rate?

8. Ordered: 1000 ml 0.9% saline to infuse at 40 gtt/min. Drop factor is 15 gtt/ml.
   - How long will it take to infuse?

9. Ordered: 100 ml with 1 g Cephalin to infuse in 30 minutes by microdrip.
   - What is the gtt/min?

10. Ordered: 200 ml to infuse at 50 gtt/min. Drop factor is microdrip.
   - How long will it take to infuse?

Worksheet   (Answers on p. 226)

Definition

Hyperalimentation or total parenteral nutrition (TPN) is the intravenous delivery of nourishment. Protein, carbohydrates, trace minerals, vitamins, and electrolytes are delivered in individualized amounts. The carbohydrates are delivered in the form of glucose (D50W, D40W).

Hyperalimentation (TPN)

42 ml/hr = 1000/24 hr
83 ml/hr = 2000/24 hr
125 ml/hr = 3000/24 hr

The glucose levels of patients receiving TPN must be monitored. Half (50%) of the volume (1000 ml) is glucose (500 ml). Each g or ml of carbohydrate equals 4 calories. Therefore 500 × 4 = 2000 calories in each 1000 ml of TPN.

1. Ordered: TPN 1000 ml to be infused at 40 ml/hr. Drop factor is 20.
   - How many gtt/min?

2. Ordered: TPN 1000 ml to be infused at 80 ml/hr continuous infusion. Drop factor is 15.
   - How many ml/24 hr?
   - How many gtt/min?

3. Ordered: TPN 1000 ml to be infused at 125 ml/hr continuous infusion. Drop factor is microdrip.
   - How many ml/hr?
   - How many gtt/min?

4. Ordered: TPN 3000 ml in 24 hr. Drop factor is 60.
   - How many gtt/min?

5. Ordered: TPN 2000 ml continuous drip in 24 hr. Drop factor is 20.
   - How many ml/hr?
   - How many gtt/min?

■ Basic Intravenous Calculations Test   (Answers on p. 226)

Write the two rules or two steps *first* and then analyze your problems. Will you begin with step 1 or step 2?

1. Ordered: 3000 ml for 24 hours. Drop factor is 15. How many gtt/min?

2. Ordered: 75 ml to be infused in 45 minutes. Drop factor is 10. How many gtt/min?

3. Ordered: 1000 ml to be infused in 12 hours IV. How many gtt/min if drop factor is 12?

4. Ordered: 1200 ml to be infused in 8 hours. Drop factor is microdrip. How many gtt/min?

5. You have 2000 ml 5% D/W being infused for 24 hours. Drop factor is 10. How many gtt/min?

6. You have 1500 ml NS to infuse. Drop factor is 15. Solution is to be given over a 12-hour period. How many ml/hr? How many gtt/min?

7. You have 3000 ml 5 D/W being infused for 24 hours with 0.5 g of penicillin in each 1000 ml. Drop factor is 60, by microdrip. How many gtt/min?

8. You have 500 ml NS being infused for 6 hours. Drop factor is 15. How many gtt/min?

9. Ordered: 1000 ml to run for 12 hours on microdrip. How many gtt/min will you regulate flow?

10. Ordered: 250 ml to infuse in 90 minutes. How many gtt/min using microdrip?

CHAPTER 7

Insulin

Objectives

- Prepare single and mixed insulin dosages.
- Identify the different types of insulin and their actions.

> **RULE:** Use insulin syringes only. There are 0.5 ml or 1ml syringes.

Explanation

The value and purity of drugs from animal sources vary. Therefore some hormones, such as insulin and heparin, are supplied in *units* (U), a standardized measurement based on strength rather than weight. You already know that insulin is an aqueous solution of the active principal hormone of the pancreas. It affects the metabolism of glucose. Insulin comes from animal sources of beef and pork pancreas, and recombinant DNA techniques (Humulin).*

Insulin is supplied in units and is given with special insulin syringes. Most commonly, insulin is supplied in 10-ml vials labeled U 100, which means 100 U/ml. Insulin is also supplied in 10-ml vials labeled "U 500," which means 500 U/ml.† This strength is used for diabetic patients whose blood sugar fluctuates to very high levels. The concentrated solution of 500 U/ml allows a concentrated dose in less fluid, avoiding the pain of large fluid injections.

Because many patients require insulin injections on a regular basis, it is important to use multiple injection sites and to plan the rotation schedule (Fig. 3).

Syringes

Insulin is usually given in a 1-ml or 0.5-ml insulin syringe calibrated to U 100 insulin. The 0.5-ml insulin syringe is used for smaller doses, as the calibrations are larger and easier to read. (Fig. 4).

---

*Humulin is the most common type of insulin administered.
†For brittle diabetes.

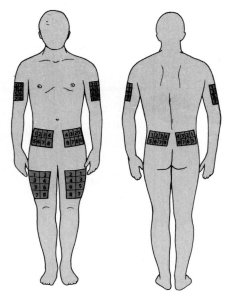

Fig. 3. Subcutaneous injection site diagram. (From Potter PA and Perry AG: Fundamentals of nursing: concepts, process, and practice, ed 2, 1989, St Louis, Mosby–Year Book.)

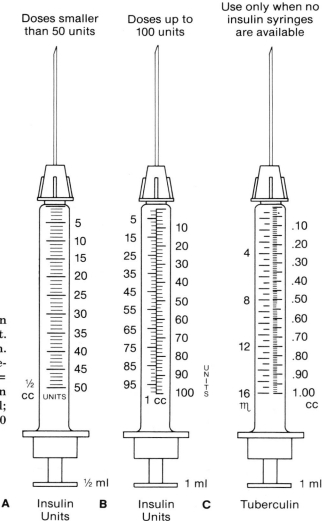

Fig. 4. Types of syringes. **A,** Insulin units. Each calibration represents 1 unit. Used for smaller doses of U-100 insulin. **B,** Insulin units. Each calibration represents 2 units. **C,** Tuberculin (16 minim = 1 ml). Minims on one side, graduated on the other side in 0.01 (hundredths) ml; 0.01 is the same as 1 unit and 0.10 ml = 10 units.

Doses smaller than 50 units

Doses up to 100 units

Use only when no insulin syringes are available

A Insulin Units   **B** Insulin Units   **C** Tuberculin

A typical order for insulin must include:
  a. The *name* of the insulin: regular, lente, NPH, etc.
  b. The *number* of units the patient will receive: regular insulin 10 U.
  c. The *time* to be given: regular insulin 10 U, in AM, ½ hr a.c.
  d. The *amount* to be given: regular insulin U 100, 10 U, in AM, ½ hr a.c.

EXAMPLE: Give 30 units of U 100 Humulin R insulin using a U 100 syringe. Fill syringe to the 30 U calibration. Always have another registered nurse check the order, label, and dosage before administering. For U 500, have *two* nurses check.

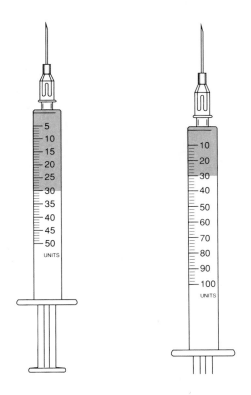

Insulin

People who need insulin are diabetics. The medical term is diabetes mellitus. A chronic deficiency of insulin is called type I (insulin-dependent) diabetes, in which the beta cells of the pancreas do not secrete any insulin. Type II diabetes (non-insulin–dependent) may be controlled by diet and oral hypoglycemics because the beta cells do supply some insulin. People who are receiving total parenteral nutrition (TPN), which is high in glucose, may also need insulin.

■ U-100. Insulin products

| | Label | Source | Onset of action | FAST-ACTING | |
				Peak (hr)	Duration (hr)
Lilly	Humulin R Regular	Human	30 min	2-5	6-8
	Iletin I R Regular	Beef/pork	15-30 min	2-5	6-8
	Iletin II R Semilente	Pork	15-30 min	2-5	5-7
	Iletin I S	Beef/pork	15-30 min	2-5	5-8
Novo Nordisk	Novolin R	Human	30 min	2-5	5-8
	Velosulin Human	Human	30 min	2-5	5-8

A

Lilly
10 mL HI-210
NDC 0002-8215-01
100 units per mL
U-100
Humulin R
REGULAR
insulin human injection, USP recombinant DNA origin

Neutral
YD 1312 AMX
Eli Lilly and Company
Indianapolis, IN 46285, U.S.A.
Keep in a cold place. Avoid freezing. If pregnant or nursing, see carton.
Important. See enclosed circular.
Exp. Date/Control No.
DISPLAY ONLY

B

10 cc   NDC 0002-8210-01   CP-210
Lilly
U-100
REGULAR ILETIN® I INSULIN INJECTION USP
100 UNITS PER CC

YC 9013 AMX
Eli Lilly AND COMPANY
Indianapolis, IN 46285, U.S.A.
KEEP IN A COLD PLACE—AVOID FREEZING. If pregnant or nursing, see carton. Made from Beef and Pork Zinc-Insulin Crystals.
Neutral
IMPORTANT—SEE WARNINGS ON ACCOMPANYING CIRCULAR
Exp. Date/Control No.
DISPLAY ONLY

C

10 cc   NDC 0002-8211-01   CP-210P
Lilly
U-100
REGULAR ILETIN® II INSULIN INJECTION USP PURIFIED PORK
100 UNITS PER CC
PORK

YC 7443 AMX
Eli Lilly AND COMPANY
Indianapolis, IN 46285, U.S.A.
KEEP IN A COLD PLACE—AVOID FREEZING. If pregnant or nursing, see carton. Made from Purified Pork Zinc-Insulin Crystals.
Neutral
IMPORTANT—SEE WARNINGS ON ACCOMPANYING CIRCULAR
Exp. Date/Control No.
DISPLAY ONLY

D

10 cc   NDC 0002-8510-01   CP-510
Lilly
U-100
SEMILENTE® ILETIN® I PROMPT INSULIN ZINC SUSPENSION USP
100 UNITS PER CC

YC 9044 AMX
Eli Lilly AND COMPANY
Indianapolis, IN 46285, U.S.A.
KEEP IN A COLD PLACE—AVOID FREEZING. If pregnant or nursing, see carton. Made from Beef and Pork Zinc-Insulin Crystals. To mix, roll or carefully shake the insulin bottle several times.
IMPORTANT—SEE WARNINGS ON ACCOMPANYING CIRCULAR
Exp. Date/Control No.
DISPLAY ONLY

E

Novolin® R
NDC 0003-1833-10
Novo Nordisk™
Regular Human Insulin Injection (semi-synthetic) USP
10 ml   100 units/ml

0604-31-102-5

For information contact:
Novo Nordisk Pharmaceuticals Inc. Princeton, NJ 08540
Manufactured by Novo Nordisk A/S DK-2880 Bagsvaerd, Denmark
Distributed by Bristol-Myers Squibb Princeton, NJ 08540
Use with **U-100** insulin syringes only See insert Keep in a cold place Avoid freezing **Change insulin only under medical supervision**
Exp. Date: Control:

F

Velosulin® Human
Regular human insulin injection (semi-synthetic)
100 units per ml · 10 ml
Novo Nordisk™

R
Human

6412-03

USE WITH U-100 SYRINGE ONLY - SEE INSERT
Warning : Do not use if the vial contents are viscous or not water clear.
CHANGE INSULIN ONLY UNDER MEDICAL SUPERVISION.
Keep in a cold place, avoid freezing.
Preservative : m-cresol 0.3%

For information contact: Novo Nordisk Pharmaceuticals Inc. Princeton, NJ 08540
Manufactured by Novo Nordisk A/S 2880 Bagsvaerd, Denmark
Distributed by Bristol - Myers Squibb Princeton, NJ 08540

NDC 0003-0111-01
NSN 6505-01-190-9248
Control No. :
Exp. date :

	Label	Source	Onset of action	INTERMEDIATE-ACTING Peak (hr)	Duration (hr)
Lilly	Humulin L	Human	1-3 hr	6-12	14-24
	Humulin N	Human	1-3 hr	6-12	14-24
	Lente Iletin I L	Beef/pork	1-2 hr	6-12	18-24
	Lente Iletin II L	Pork	1-2 hr	6-12	18-24
	NPH Iletin I N	Beef/pork	1-2 hr	6-12	18-24
	NPH Iletin II N	Pork	1-2 hr	6-12	18-24
Novo Nordisk	Novolin L	Human	2½-5 hr	7-15	18-24

G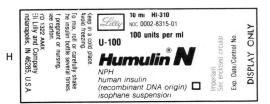

H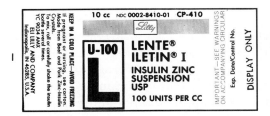

I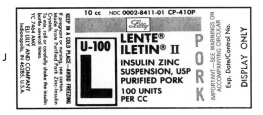

J

K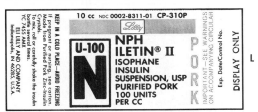

L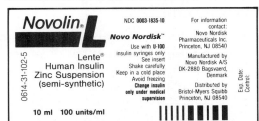

M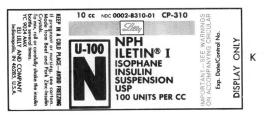

Continued.

Label	Source	Onset of action	LONG-ACTING Peak (hr)	Duration (hr)
			Long-acting	
Humulin Ultralente	Human	4-6 hr	8-20	24-28
Protamine Zinc Iletin I	Beef/pork	4-6 hr	14-24	28-36
PZI II	Pork	4-6 hr	14-24	28-36
Ultralente Iletin I	Beef/pork	4-6 hr	14-24	28-36

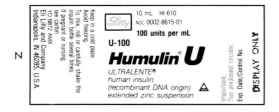

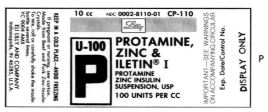

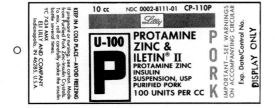

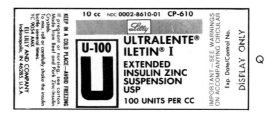

Mixing Insulins

Insulin dosages are drawn up *exactly* as ordered. An incorrect dosage could be devastating to the patient. Frequently, regular or fast-acting insulin is combined with an intermediate-acting insulin. This gives insulin coverage (glucose control) within 15 to 20 minutes and lasts 15 to 24 hours. This technique of combining the two types of insulin is important for the nurse, patient, and family to master. The regular insulin vial should *not* be contaminated with the longer-acting insulin.

> RULE: When mixing insulins, remember that only the same species or sources can be mixed, such as pork and pork or beef/pork and beef/pork or human and human.

RULE:	Mix only those insulins which have the same strength, such as U-100 with U-100.

Read orders correctly. Dosage errors are made by misinterpreting the order.

EXAMPLE: 5 U may be misread as 50 units.

The most common complication of insulin therapy is hypoglycemia, which may be caused by injecting too much insulin (at home risk), not eating enough, or exercising too much.

EXAMPLE: All problems use U-100 strength.

ORDERED: 10 units of Regular Iletin I and 20 units of NPH Iletin I. Refer to p. 104-106 for labels and source.

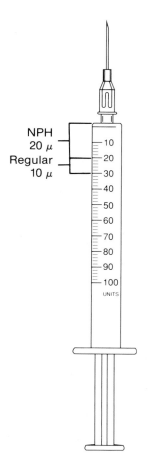

Total units: 30

Onset/Duration: 15 min-24 hr

Peak: 2-12 hr

Labels: B and K

Source: Beef/pork and beef/pork

Which insulin will you draw up first? ____B____

Reading syringes correctly

1. Units measured: _____

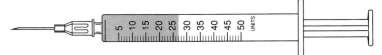

2. Units measured: _____

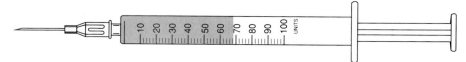

3. Units measured: _____

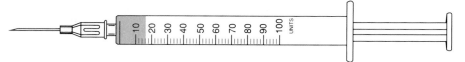

4. Units measured: _____

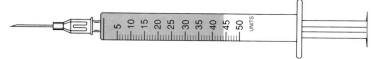

5. Units measured: _____

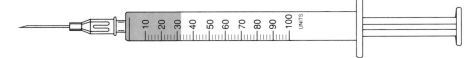

6. Units measured: _____

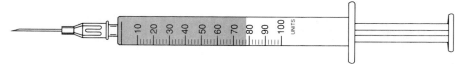

Worksheet   (Answers on p. 227)

Shade syringe to match your dosage of each type of insulin and label. Fill in the blanks next to each statement as shown in the example.

1.   Ordered: 20 units of Semilente I and 35 units of Lente I ½ hr a.c. breakfast.

Total units: _____
Onset/duration: _____
Peak: _____
Labels: _____
Which drawn up first: _____
Source: _____

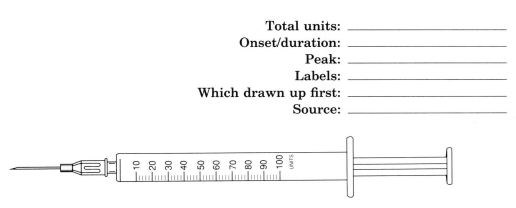

2.   Ordered: Humulin R 18 units and Humulin N 25 units.

Total units: _____
Onset/duration: _____
Peak: _____
Labels: _____
Source: _____

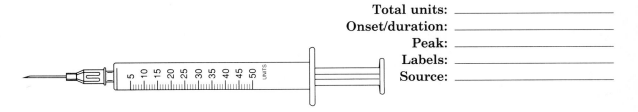

3.   Ordered: Iletin II R 8 units and Iletin II NPH 15 units.

Total units: _____
Onset/duration: _____
Peak: _____
Labels: _____
Source: _____

4. Ordered: Iletin I R 22 units and Iletin II NPH 35 units.

Total units: _____
Onset/duration: _____
Peak: _____
Labels: _____
Source: _____

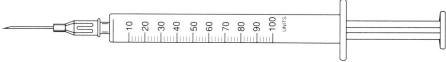

5. Ordered: Iletin I Regular insulin 8 units and Iletin I NPH I 60 units ½ hr a.c. breakfast.

Total units: _____
Onset/duration: _____
Peak: _____
Labels: _____
Source: _____

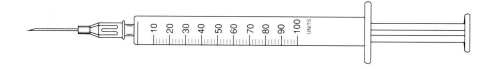

6. Ordered: Humulin R 10 units and Humulin N 40 units ½ hr a.c. breakfast.

Total units: _____
Onset/duration: _____
Peak: _____
Labels: _____
Source: _____

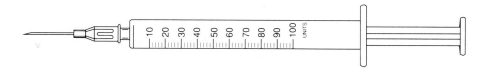

7. Ordered: Regular Iletin II 14 units and Lente Iletin II 32 units.

Total units: _____
Onset/duration: _____
Peak: _____
Labels: _____
Source: _____

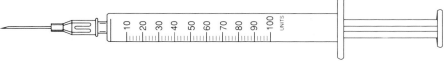

8. Ordered: ½ hour a.c. breakfast give Semilente Iletin I 18 units and NPH Iletin I 46 units.

Total units: _____
Onset/duration: _____
Peak: _____
Label: _____
Source: _____

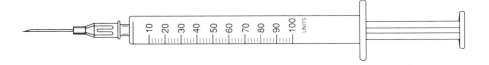

9. Ordered: Novolin R 7 units and Novolin L 35 units.

Total units: _____
Onset/duration: _____
Peak: _____
Label: _____
Source: _____

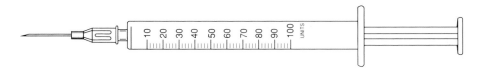

10. Ordered: Velosulin Human 20 units and Humulin N 56 units ½ hr a.c. breakfast.

Total units: _____

Onset/duration: _____

Peak: _____

Label: _____

Source: _____

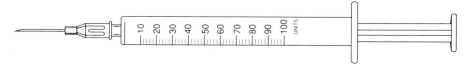

7C **Worksheet**   (Answers on p. 228)

Shade in insulin amounts on syringes. Refer to insulin chart on p. 104-106 for onset, peak, and duration.

1. You are to give 35 units of Humulin R insulin. You have a bottle labeled regular insulin U 100. How many units will you measure? Shade in the amount you will give.

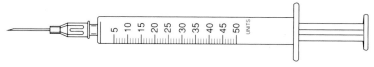

2. Ordered: 20 units of Humulin R insulin a.c. t.i.d. On hand: regular insulin. How many units will you give? _____ When will the action begin (onset)? _____

3. Ordered: Lente I L 44 units qd. On hand: Lente I L. How many units will you give? _____ When will it peak? _____

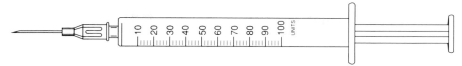

4. Ordered: Regular Iletin I insulin 65 units. Available: regular insulin Iletin I. How many units will you give? _____ How long will the action last? _____

5. Ordered: 20 units of Iletin II regular insulin stat. Available: regular Iletin II insulin. You will give _____ units. When will the action begin (onset)? _____

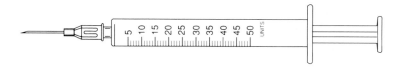

6. Ordered: Humulin R 20 units and Humulin L 40 units SC every AM ½ a.c. How many total units will you give? _____ What is the onset/duration? _____

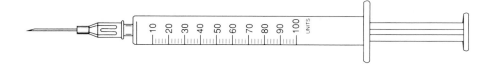

7. Ordered: Iletin I regular insulin 15 units. Available: Iletin I regular insulin U 100. You will give _____ units. Who will check your dosage? _____

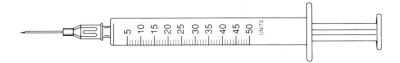

8. Ordered: Ultralente I 30 units SC. When will this peak? _____ What is the duration? _____

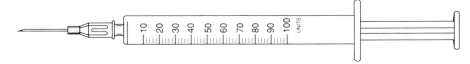

9. Ordered: Semilente insulin 25 units SC qAM. What is the onset? _____ What is the peak? _____

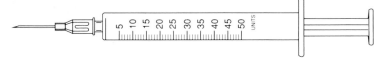

10. Ordered: Ultralente insulin 30 units qAM. What is the peak? _____ What is the duration? _____

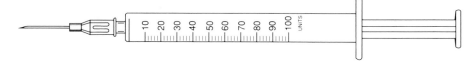

Intravenous Insulin

Explanation

During acute phases of illness, insulin is given by the intravenous route to ensure a controlled supply of medication that will vary depending on laboratory monitoring. Infusion is usually administered with an IMED or IV pump. To prevent insulin from being absorbed by the plastic infusion bag, albumin may be added.

> **RULE:** Begin the problem with known amount of medication in the total solution.

EXAMPLE: ORDERED: Regular insulin* 5 U/hr IV drip. Pharmacy has delivered 100 ml 0.9% NS with 100 U regular insulin.

- How many ml/hr will infuse 5 U/hr?
- How many hours will the IV infuse?
- How many gtt/min will infuse 5 U/hr?

	Have	**Want to know**

Step 1: 100 U:100 ml::5 U:x ml   PROOF: $100 \times 5 = 500$

$100x = 100 \times 5 = 500$ $100 \times 5 = 500$

$100x = 500$

$x = 5$ ml/hr $= 5$ U of insulin $= 5$ gtt/min

	Know	**Want to know**

Step 2: 5 ml:1 hr::100 ml:x hr   PROOF: $20 \times 5 = 100$

$5x = 100$ $1 \times 100 = 100$

$x = 20$

---

*Only regular insulin can be used intravenously.

Worksheet   (Answers on p. 229)

For the following problems, answer:

- gtt/min to infuse the units/hr with microdrip tubing
- ml/hr to infuse the ordered amount
- length of time IV is to infuse

1. Ordered: 100 U Regular Humulin insulin IV at 10 U/hr. You have 150 ml of 0.9% NS with 100 U Humulin regular insulin.

2. Ordered: 50 ml 0.9% NS with 50 U Humulin regular insulin. Infuse at 8 U/hr.

3. Ordered: 50 ml 0.9% NS with 75 U Humulin regular insulin to infuse at 5 U/hr.

4. Ordered: 120 U Humulin regular insulin IV at 10 U/hr. You have 100 ml of NS 0.9% with 120 U Humulin regular insulin.

5. Ordered: 150 U Humulin regular insulin IV at 12 U/hr. You have 150 ml of NS 0.9% with 150 U of Humulin regular insulin.

6. Ordered: 50 U Humulin regular insulin to infuse in 24 hr. Pharmacy has sent 500 ml 0.9% NS with 50 U Humulin of regular insulin.

7. Ordered: 100 U Humulin regular insulin in 250 ml 0.9% NS to infuse in 24 hours.

8. Ordered: 100 U of Humulin regular insulin in 50 ml 0.9% NS to infuse in 24 hours.

9. Ordered: 25 U Humulin regular insulin to infuse in 12 hours. Pharmacy has sent 100 ml 0.9% NS with 25 U of Humulin regular insulin.

10. Ordered: 65 U Humulin regular insulin to infuse in 24 hours. You have 65 U in 150 ml of 0.9% NS.

Madison, John   Rm 302
Age: 54   Dr. Jones
41-202-90-6

MEDICATION ADMINISTRATION RECORD

DATE	DRUG DOSE ROUTE		DATE DC	TIME SCHEDULE	DATE 9/5			DATE			DATE		
					11-7	7-3	3-11	11-7	7-3	3-11	11-7	7-3	3-11
9/5	*Insulin Check Order*	IM IV PO R SC											
		IM IV PO R SC											
		IM IV PO R SC											
		IM IV PO R SC											
		IM IV PO R SC											
		IM IV PO R SC											
		IM IV PO R SC											
		IM IV PO R SC											
		IM IV PO R SC											
		IM IV PO R SC											
		IM IV PO R SC											
		IM IV PO R SC											
		IM IV PO R SC											
		IM IV PO R SC											
		IM IV PO R SC											
		IM IV PO R SC											
		IM IV PO R SC											
		IM IV PO R SC											

PRN/ONE TIME ONLY ORDERS

	IM IV PO R SC											
	IM IV PO R SC											
	IM IV PO R SC											
	IM IV PO R SC											
	IM IV PO R SC											
	IM IV PO R SC											
	IM IV PO R SC											
	IM IV PO R SC											

KEY							Signature	Initials	Signature	Initials	Signature	Initials
ABD - ABDOMEN		**O** - NOT GIVEN		**RA** - RT. ARM								
LA - LT. ARM		**OD** - RT. EYE		**RT** - RT. THIGH								
LT - LT. THIGH		**OS** - LT. EYE		**RU** - RUQ								
IVPB - IV PIGGYBACK			**SQ** - SUBCUTANEOUS									

LU - LUQ   **OU** - BOTH EYES

ALLERGIES
   NKA

■ Insulin Test   (Answers on p. 232)

Shade in amounts on insulin.

Carry out to two decimal places (hundredths):

1. Ordered: Humulin regular insulin 65 U stat. Available: regular insulin U 100. How many units will you give?

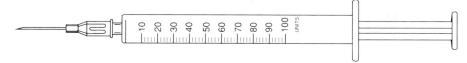

2. Ordered: Humulin regular insulin 5 U. Available: regular insulin U 100. How many units will you give?

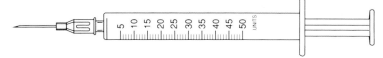

3. Ordered: Iletin I regular insulin 16 U with Iletin I NPH insulin 30 U. Available: Iletin I U 100. Shade in units of regular insulin. Shade in amount of NPH.

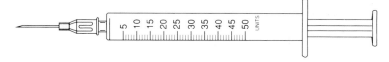

4. Ordered: Lente insulin 18 U qd. How many units will you give?

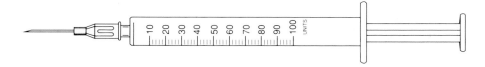

5. Ordered: Humulin Lente insulin 46 U and Humulin R 18 U. How many total units will you give?

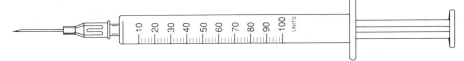

6. Ordered: 10 U/hr Humulin R regular insulin IV. Pharmacy sent 500 ml 0.9% saline with 250 U Humulin R regular insulin.
   - How many hours will the IV infuse?
   - How many ml/hr will deliver 10 U/hr?

7. Ordered: 6 U/hr Humulin R regular insulin. You have a 10-ml vial of U 100 Humulin R regular insulin and 250 ml of 0.9% saline. You add 100 U Humulin R of regular insulin (1 ml).
   - How many ml/hr will infuse 6 U of insulin?
   - How many hours will the infusion last?

8. Ordered: 8 U/hr Humulin R regular insulin IV. Pharmacy has sent 250 ml NS with 100 U insulin.
   - How many ml/hr will infuse?
   - How many hours will the IV infuse?

9. Ordered: 7 U/hr regular Iletin I insulin IV. Pharmacy has sent 200 ml NS with 100 U Iletin I regular insulin.
   - How many ml/hr will infuse 7 U/hr?
   - How many hours will the IV infuse?

10. Ordered: Semilente Iletin I regular insulin 9 U/hr IV. Pharmacy sent 500 ml NS with 100 U Semilente Iletin I insulin.
    - How many ml/hr will infuse 9 U/hr?
    - How many hours will the IV infuse?

CHAPTER 8

Heparin

Objectives

- Convert heparin units to hundredths or tenths of a milliliter.
- Calculate IV heparin units and ml/hr.

Explanation

Sodium heparin injection, USP, is a drug used to interrupt the clotting process. It may be given in therapeutic dosages or in small diluted dosages to maintain the patency of IV or IA lines. Because it is inactive orally, sodium heparin is usually administered intravenously or subcutaneously. If administered intramuscularly, the drug produces a high level of pain and may cause hematomas. Sodium heparin is obtained commercially from domestic animals slaughtered for food. The orders for heparin are highly individualized and based on laboratory studies. Heparin comes in various strengths, including 5000 U/ml, 10,000 U/ml, 20,000 U/ml, and 50,000 U/ml.

The vial must be checked carefully before administration. Heparin is fast acting and may be counteracted with protamine sulfate. Check laboratory values for clotting times *before* administering heparin. Heparin orders, dosage, vial, and amount in syringe should be checked with another registered nurse. Heparin must not be interrupted and is incompatible with other medications.

Heparin is supplied in units, as is insulin, because the purity varies among sources. Heparin is often supplied in preprepared syringes. If you need to give less than the amount in the syringe, calculate the fractional amount you need to give and then transfer the heparin to a tuberculin syringe.*

RULE:	The dosage of SC heparin should not exceed 1 ml.

---

*The new syringe with sterile needle is advisable because the heparin inside the original needle may track through the subcutaneous tissue on insertion and cause bruising. Add 0.2 ml of air to syringe to ensure that all medication is administered, which will prevent tracking.

EXAMPLE: ORDERED: Heparin 3500 U SC. On hand is a prepared vial containing 5000 U/ml. How many ml will you give?

Have   **Want**

5000 U:1 ml::3500 U:x ml

$5000x = 3500$

$x = 0.7$ ml

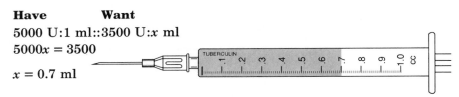

|8A| **Worksheet**   (Answers on p. 233)

SUBCUTANEOUS INJECTIONS

If a multiple-dose vial is used, choose the strength that ensures that less than 1 ml will be injected. Label and prove, shading in dosage on syringe (carry out to nearest hundredths).

1.   Give heparin 7000 U. On hand you have heparin 10,000 U/ml. How many ml will you give?

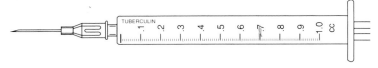

2.   Ordered: 15,000 U heparin. How many ml will you give if you have heparin 20,000 U/ml?

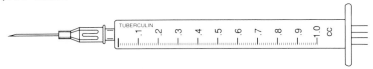

3. Ordered: heparin 2500 U. On hand you have heparin 20,000 U/ml. How many ml will you give?

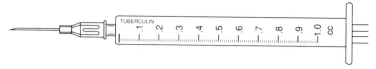

4. Ordered: heparin 17,000 U. On hand you have heparin 10,000 U/ml and 20,000 U/ml. Which strength will you choose? How many ml will you give?

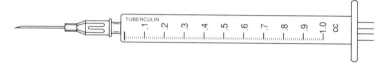

5. Ordered: heparin 7500 U. How many ml will you give if the vial on hand reads heparin 10,000 U/ml?

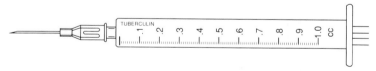

Worksheet   (Answers on p. 234)

The heparin will be administered with an infusion pump.

1. Ordered: heparin sodium 1000 U/hr IV. Pharmacy has sent 1 L of 0.9% saline with 20,000 U of heparin. How many ml/hr will deliver 1000 U?

2. Ordered: heparin sodium 20,000 U IV in 12 hours. Pharmacy has sent 1000 ml with 20,000 U heparin sodium. How many ml/hr should the IV infuse? How many U/hr will infuse?

3. Ordered: heparin 1500 U/hr IV. Pharmacy has sent 1 L 0.9% saline with 20,000 U of heparin. How many ml/hr will deliver 1500 U?

4. Ordered: heparin 10,000 U in 15 hours. Pharmacy has sent 1000 ml NS with 10,000 U of heparin. How many U/hr will the patient receive? How many ml/hr will be infused?

5. Ordered: heparin 1200 U/hr. Pharmacy has sent 500 ml NS with 10,000 U of heparin. How many ml/hr will infuse 1200 U/hr?

6. Ordered: heparin 2000 U/hr IV. You have 50,000 U per 1000 ml 0.9% NS. How many ml/hr will deliver 2,000 U/hr?

7. Ordered: heparin 1000 U/hr IV. Pharmacy delivered 25,000 U/500 ml. How many ml/hr will deliver 1000 U/hr?

8. Ordered: heparin 1,300 U/hr IV. You have 500 ml with 25,000 U of heparin sodium. How many ml/hr will deliver 1,300 U/hr?

9. Ordered: 1800 U/hr of heparin IV. Your patient is on fluid restrictions, therefore the pharmacy has sent a concentrated solution of 25,000 U/250 ml of NS. How many ml/hr will deliver 1800 U/hr?

10. Ordered: 1000 U/hr heparin IV. Your patient is on fluid restrictions. Pharmacy has sent 20,000 U/250 ml of NS. How many ml/hr will deliver 1000 U/hr?

Patrick, John   Rm 401 B
Age:
02/05/13   Dr. Killian

MEDICATION ADMINISTRATION RECORD

DATE	DRUG DOSE ROUTE		DATE DC	TIME SCHEDULE	DATE 10/15			DATE 10/16			DATE		
					11-7	7-3	3-11	11-7	7-3	3-11	11-7	7-3	3-11
10/15	Heparin 500 u	IM IV PO R (SC)		q 6h	0600 ABD KR	1200 ABD KR	1800 ABD KR	2400 ABD KR					
		IM IV PO R SC											
		IM IV PO R SC											
		IM IV PO R SC											
		IM IV PO R SC											
		IM IV PO R SC											
		IM IV PO R SC											
		IM IV PO R SC											
		IM IV PO R SC											
		IM IV PO R SC											
		IM IV PO R SC											
		IM IV PO R SC											
		IM IV PO R SC											
		IM IV PO R SC											
		IM IV PO R SC											
		IM IV PO R SC											
		IM IV PO R SC											
		IM IV PO R SC											

PRN/ONE TIME ONLY ORDERS

		IM IV PO R SC											
		IM IV PO R SC											
		IM IV PO R SC											
		IM IV PO R SC											
		IM IV PO R SC											
		IM IV PO R SC											
		IM IV PO R SC											

KEY				Signature	Initials	Signature	Initials	Signature	Initials
ABD - ABDOMEN	**O** - NOT GIVEN	**RA** - RT. ARM		Kay Rae	KR				
LA - LT. ARM	**OD** - RT. EYE	**RT** - RT. THIGH							
LT - LT. THIGH	**OS** - LT. EYE	**RU** - RUQ							

LU - LUQ   **OU** - BOTH EYES

IVPB - IV PIGGYBACK   **SQ** - SUBCUTANEOUS

ALLERGIES Penicillin

■ 126

■ Heparin Test   (Answers on p. 236)

1. Ordered: heparin 4000 U SC. The vial on hand is 5000 U/ml. How many ml will you give using a TB syringe?

2. Ordered: heparin 2500 U q4h SC. The vial on hand is labeled 10,000 U/ml. How many ml will you give using a TB syringe?

3. Ordered: 2000 U heparin q4h SC. The vials on hand are 5000 U/ml and 10,000 U/ml. Which vial will you choose? Using a tuberculin syringe, how many ml will you give?

4. Ordered: 7000 U heparin q6h SC. The vials on hand are 5000 U/ml, 10,000 U/ml, and 20,000 U/ml. Which one will you choose? How many ml will you give?

5. Ordered: 3000 U heparin q4h SC. On hand is a vial of heparin 5000 U/ml. Using a tuberculin syringe, how many ml will you give?

6. Ordered: 700 U/hr IV. You have 20,000 U/500 ml. How many ml/hr will provide 700 U/hr?

7. Ordered: 1500 U/hr IV. You have 25,000 U/500 ml. How many ml/hr will provide 1500 U/hr?

8. Ordered: 25,000 U heparin IV in 24 hrs. You have 1000 ml with 25,000 U of heparin sodium. How many ml/hr will give 25,000 U in 24 hr? How many U/hr will infuse?

9. Ordered: heparin 1800 U/hr. Pharmacy has sent you 500 ml 0.9% NS with 25,000 U of heparin sodium. How many ml/hr will deliver 1800 U/hr?

10. You are working in a clinic and giving PPD (TB) intradermal injections for TB screening. How much will you draw up in the syringe? Indicate the amount you will give on the syringe.

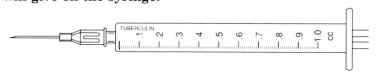

CHAPTER 9

Children's dosages

Objectives

- Estimate kilograms for given number of pounds.

- Calculate kilograms for given number of pounds and ounces.

- Calculate 24-hour doses.

- Calculate safe dose ranges in milligrams and micrograms per kilogram and stated weight in pounds and ounces.

- Calculate pediatric doses using BSA formula.

- Determine if pediatric drug order is within safe dose range.

Explanation

Babies and children should receive less medication than adults. It is very important for the nurse to double-check all physicians' medication orders for children and infants with written reliable references to be certain that the dose ordered is within the safe range recommended by the literature.

Prompt clarification with the physician is important if the dose is too low to be therapeutic or represents an overdose.

The two methods currently used for calculating safe pediatric doses are based on (1) body weight in milligrams or micrograms per kilogram of body weight (mg/kg or µg/kg), and on (2) body surface area (BSA) in square meters (m^2) using a scale called a *nomogram.**

Mg/kg method

The mg/kg method is the most frequently used means of calculating a therapeutic dose for pediatric medication administration. The literature accompanying most medications states the safe amount of drug in milligrams per kilogram of body weight, usually for a 24-hour period. The amount of mg/kg is less for children than for adults. You may also see µg/kg cited for therapeutic dose when very small amounts of medication will be given.

---

*See the Appendix, p. 176, for examples of formulas used to estimate pediatric doses when literature is unavailable.

> **RULE:** Calculate the safe dose range cited in the literature using the current body weight of the child. Compare and evaluate the results with the physician's 24-hour order.*

Steps to solving problems

1. Estimate the child's weight in kg by dividing the pounds in half (12 lb = approximately 6 kg). Always estimate your answers.
2. Calculate the child's exact weight in kg to the nearest tenth (45.18 = 45.2 kg).† Note whether this calculation will be a one-step or two-step problem.
   a. If the child's weight is in ounces (for example, 8 lb, 6 oz), first convert the ounces to nearest tenth of a pound. Add this to the pounds which will give total weight. Then convert the pounds (total) to kilograms. (This would be a two-step calculation.)
   b. If the child's weight is already in pounds only (for example, 8 lb), convert the pounds to kg. (This would be a one-step calculation.) Safety check: Is your answer close to the estimate?
3. Consult the literature for the safe pediatric range for this medication in mg/kg or μg/kg. Set up a ratio and proportion with the recommended mg/kg as the known and the x = mg/child's weight in kg as the amount you want to know.
4. Compare and evaluate the 24-hour ordered amount with the recommended safe amount determined by your calculations.‡ Make a decision to **Give** (safe dose), **Give and clarify** (underdose), or **Hold and clarify** promptly (overdose).

EXAMPLE: Ordered: Lincocin 50 mg q6h IM. Baby weighs 12 lb, 6 oz today. On hand you have Lincocin 300 mg/ml. The literature states that the safe range is 20 mg/kg q24h.§

- What is the estimated weight in kg?
  12 ÷ 2 = 6 kg estimated weight

- What is the exact weight in kg? A weight of 12 lb, 6 oz involves a two-step conversion.

---

*Be sure the two comparisons are for the same time periods.
†See p. 24 for instructions on rounding.
‡Use written literature for medication references.
§The literature now cites mg/kg or mg/m^2 for most medications for children.

Know   **Want to know**

a.   16 oz:1 lb::6 oz:x lb

$$\frac{16x}{16} = \frac{6}{16} = 0.37 \text{ or } 0.4 \text{ lb}$$

PROOF: $16 \times 0.37 = 5.92$ or 6
           $1 \times 6 = 6$

Baby weighs 12.4 lb.

Know   **Want to know**

b.   2.2 lb:1 kg::12.4 lb:x kg

$$\frac{2.2x}{2.2} = \frac{12.4}{2.2} = 5.62$$

PROOF: $2.2 \times 5.62 = 12.4$
           $1 \times 12.4 = 12.4$

Baby weighs 5.6 kg.

■ What is the recommended dose for this child's weight?

Know   **Want to know**

20 mg:1 kg::x mg:5.6 kg

$x = 112$ mg (safe 24-hour dose)

PROOF: $20 \times 5.6 = 112$
           $1 \times 112 = 112$

■ Is the order safe to give?
No.

Order is 50 mg × 4, or 200 mg for 24 hours. The order exceeds the recommended dose. Hold and clarify stat. Document. Unsafe order.

BSA method (mg/m^2)

The body surface area (BSA) method is the most reliable way to calculate therapeutic dosages. It requires the use of a chart (nomogram; Fig. 5) that converts weight to square meters (m^2) of BSA. The average adult is assumed to weigh 140 lb and have 1.7 m^2 BSA. The BSA method is usually used to calculate safe doses for antineoplastic drugs,* new drugs, or drugs that normally aren't given to children. It is also used to determine therapeutic doses for underweight or overweight persons.

> **RULE:**   To determine the BSA (m^2) of a child of normal height for weight, find the m^2 for that weight on the appropriate nomogram (Fig. 5).

---

*With antineoplastic therapy, doses are individualized on the basis of the severity of the illness, the liver and renal function of the child, the response to therapy, individual versus multiple-dose therapy, and the sequence of the dose (first dose or later doses). Some doses for young children approach adult doses. Some tumors are now treated aggressively with "megadoses"—very large doses. When in doubt, clarify with the physician and document.

EXAMPLE: A child weighs 10 lb. Using the nomogram column for children of normal height for weight, a 10-lb child has a BSA of 0.27 m^2 (Fig. 5, A).

EXAMPLE: A girl weighs 25 lb and is 32 inches (normal height for her weight). According to the nomogram (Fig. 5, A) for children of normal height for weight, the BSA for 25 lb is 0.52.

RULE: To determine the BSA (m^2) of a child who is underweight or over-weight, find the m^2 for that weight by plotting the height in the height column and the weight in the weight column, using a straight line to join the two numbers. Where the line intersects on the surface area (SA) column is the m^2 for that child.

EXAMPLE: A 9 lb, 14 oz baby with a height of 60 cm would be underweight for height. Using a ruler to connect his height and weight, you would find a BSA of 0.28 m^2 (Fig. 5, B) in the SA column.

Steps to solving mg/m^2 problems*

1. Check doctor's order and check recommended dose in literature.

   Ordered: 15 mg prednisone stat
   Literature: 40 mg/m^2 for children with Hodgkin's disease

2. Determine weight and height of child. Consult the appropriate nomogram (Fig. 5) and columns to obtain BSA in m^2.

   9.1 kg or 22.75 lb with normal height of 71 cm.
   BSA is approximately 0.48 m^2.

3. Calculate the recommended mg/m^2 dose in the literature using ratio and pro-portion (as you did with the mg/kg method), and compare it with the dose ordered for safety (recommended mg:1 m^2::x mg::child's m^2).

   Know   **Want to know**
   40 mg:1 m^2::x mg:0.48 m^2
   $x = 40 \times 0.48$
   $x = 19.20$ mg safe dose limit
   15 mg ordered
   Order is safe.

---

*The literature now cites mg/kg or mg/m^2 for most medications for children.

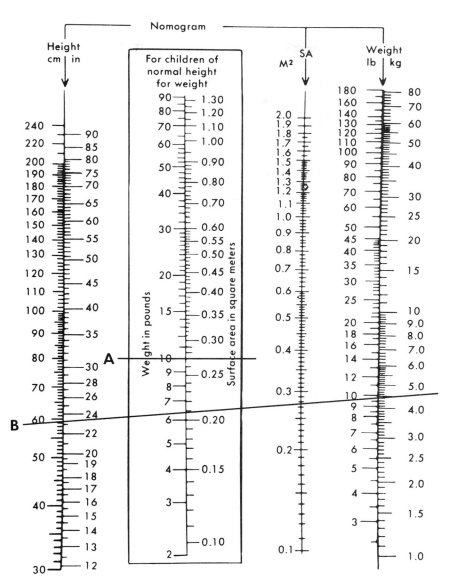

Fig. 5. West nomogram (for estimation of surface areas). **A,** When the child is normal height for weight, use the enclosed area for determining the body surface area (BSA). **B,** For a child who is under- or overweight, the surface area is indicated where a straight line connecting the height and weight intersects the surface areas (SA) column. (Nomogram modified from data of Boyd E by West CD: from Shirkey HC: Drug therapy. In Vaugn VC III and McKay RJ, editors: Nelson's textbook of pediatrics, ed 10, Philadelphia, 1975, WB Saunders Co.)

EXAMPLE: A 10-lb child has an m² of 0.27, and the average adult dose of a new antibiotic is 250 mg. How many mg would be safe for the child?

$$\frac{0.27}{1.7 \ m^2} \times 250 = 39.7 \text{ mg or } 40 \text{ mg}$$

EXAMPLE: A 26-lb child has an m² of 0.52, and the average adult dose of a tranquilizer is 15 mg. How many mg would be safe for the child?

$$\frac{0.52}{1.7 \ m^2} \times 15 = 4.5 \text{ mg}$$

---

*Calculate kilograms to the nearest tenth.

Worksheet (Answers on p. 237)

1. Estimate the following weights in kg. Then convert lb to kg using the ratio and proportion method. Round to the *nearest* tenth.* Prove your answer.
   a. 14 lb (1 or 2 steps?)
   b. 12 lb, 2 oz (1 or 2 steps?)
   c. 10 lb
   d. 7 lb, 6 oz
   e. 15 lb, 8 oz

2. Calculate the 24-hour total dosage in mg.
   a. 150 mg q8h
   b. 200 mg q6h
   c. 400 µg q4h
   d. 50 mg tid
   e. 750 µg q12h

3. Calculate the safe dose ranges in mg for the following weights. Use ratio and proportion.
   a. 10 mg/kg; weight is 5 kg
   b. 5-8 mg/kg; weight is 7.3 kg
   c. 6-8 mg/kg; weight is 8 lb
   d. 3-6 mg/kg; weight is 5 lb, 8 oz
   e. 200-400 µg/kg; weight is 4 lb, 6 oz

---

*For rounding instructions refer to p. 24. Round pounds and kg to *nearest* tenth.

4. State the BSA in m² for the following children of normal height and weight.*
   a. 4 lb
   b. 6 lb
   c. 10 lb
   d. 30 lb
   e. 70 lb

5. State the approximate safe dose in mg for children with the following m² using the BSA formula† and the following adult doses. Round to the nearest whole number.

	Child m²	Adult dose	BSA formula Approximate safe dose
a.	.28	125 mg	_____
b.	.32	250 mg	_____
c.	.45	5 mg	_____
d.	.80	500 mg	_____
e.	1.27	100 mg	_____

---

*Calculate kg and pounds to nearest tenth.
†For m², refer to BSA formula on p. 134.

Worksheet (Answers on p. 241)

Compare the safe-dose range with the order for a 24-hour period and make a
decision: Give (within safe dose range)
  Give and clarify (underdose)
  Hold and clarify promptly (overdose)

1. Weight: 25.4 lbs
   Order: 100 mg tid
   Reference: 10-30 mg/kg/day in divided doses

   Weight in kg*:   (kg est:)
   Recommended dose—24 hours:
   Ordered dose—24 hours:
   Decision:

2. Weight: 33 lbs
   Order: 0.5 mg tid
   Reference: 100-200 μg/kg/day in divided doses†

   Weight in kg: (kg est:)
   Recommended dose—24 hours:
   Ordered dose—24 hours:
   Decision:

*Calculate lb and kg to nearest tenth. Refer to p. 24 for rounding instructions. (Don't forget to estimate
weight in kilograms.)
†1000 μg = 1 mg

3. Weight: 20 lb
   Order: 50 mg daily
   Reference: 2-4 mg/kg/day

   Weight in kg: (kg est:)
   Recommended dose—24 hours:
   Ordered dose—24 hours:
   Decision:

4. Weight: 5 lb
   Order: 0.03 mg qid
   Reference: 10-20 μg/kg/day

   Weight in kg: (kg est:)
   Recommended dose—24 hours:
   Ordered dose—24 hours:
   Decision:

5. Weight: 85 lb
   Order: 100 mg q6h
   Reference: 10-15 mg/kg/day in divided doses

   Weight in kg: (kg est:)
   Recommended dose—24 hours:
   Ordered dose—24 hours:
   Decision:

Worksheet   (Answers on p. 243)

Children's oral medications

For each problem, calculate child's weight in kg* if required, calculate safe dose range, and compare it with the order.

Make decision: 1.   Give (within safe dose range)
                           2.   Give and clarify (underdose)
                           3.   Hold and clarify promptly (overdose)

For decisions 1 and 2, calculate medication amount† to be administered.

1.   Ordered: Dilantin 30 mg tid po for a 2-year-old child weighing 39.6 lb today. Safe dose for this age group is 5 mg/kg/day. On hand is Dilantin Pediatric Suspension 125 mg/5 ml.

2.   Ordered: ampicillin 200 mg po q6h for a baby who weighs 12 lb, 4 oz today. Safe pediatric dosage is 100 to 200 mg/kg in divided doses for 24 hours. On hand is 125 mg/5 ml ampicillin oral suspension, USP.

---

*Calculate kg to nearest tenth. Refer to p. 24 for rounding instructions.
†For amounts of less than 1 ml, calculate to nearest hundredth. For amounts of more than 1 ml, calculate to nearest tenth.

3. Ordered: mephobarbital 300 mg po q8h for a 62-lb child. Literature reads: child po 6 to 12 mg/kg/day in divided doses q6 to 8h. On hand are 100 mg tablets.

4. Ordered: paraaminosalicylate 2 g po tid for a 50-lb child. Literature reads: child po 240 to 360 mg/kg/day in 3 or 4 divided doses. On hand you have 0.5 g tablets.

5. Ordered: prednisone 20 mg/day po. The child weighs 30 lb and has normal height for weight. Safe dose for children is 40 mg/m^2/day po. Use the BSA nomogram* to determine the m^2 for this child's weight. On hand are 10 mg tablets.

*Use the West nomogram (Fig. 5, p. 133) and administer if order is not an overdose.

Worksheet   (Answers on p. 246)

Children's intramuscular medications

For each problem, calculate safe dose range and compare it with the order for same time period.

Make decision: 1.   Give (within safe dose range)
2.   Give and clarify (underdose)
3.   Hold and clarify promptly (overdose)

For decisions 1 and 2 only, calculate medication amount* to be administered.

1.   Ordered: ampicillin 75 mg q8h IM. Baby weighs 5 lb, 10 oz today.† Safe range for babies weighing less than 20 kg is 50 mg/kg in divided doses for 24 hours. On hand is 125 mg/5 ml.

2.   Ordered: lincocin 40 mg IM bid. Child weighs 9 lb, 2 oz today. Literature states for children: 20 mg/kg q12h IM. On hand is lincomycin hydrochloride 300 mg/ml.

---

*For amounts of less than 1 ml, calculate to nearest hundredth. For amounts of more than 1 ml, calculate to nearest tenth.
†Calculate pounds and kilograms to nearest tenth.

3. Ordered: Garamycin IM 20 mg tid. The child weighs 18 lb. Literature states for children: 2 to 2.5 mg/kg/q8h. On hand is 10 mg/ml Garamycin Pediatric Injectable.

4. Ordered: meperidine (Demerol) 15 mg IM preoperatively for a child who weighs 20 lb, 8 oz. Safe range for children is 1 to 2.2 mg/kg IM. On hand you have a tubex with 25 mg/ml.

5. Ordered: doxycycline hydrate 20 mg bid IM for a 40-lb child. Literature reads: 2.2 to 4.4 mg/kg/day. On hand is 50 mg/ml.

Worksheet   (Answers on p. 248)

Childrens' intravenous medications

For each problem, calculate safe dose range and compare it with the order for same time period.

Make decision: 1. Give (within safe dose range)

                  2. Give and clarify (underdose)

                  3. Hold and clarify promptly (overdose)

For decisions 1 and 2 only, calculate medication amount* to be administered.

1. Ordered: phenobarbital sodium 10 mg IV q6h. Baby's weight today is 7 lb, 2 oz. Safe range in the literature is 3 to 6 mg/kg q24h. On hand is phenobarbital sodium injectable 65 mg/ml.

2. Ordered: furosemide (Lasix) 150 mg IV. The literature states that the therapeutic range for children is 1 mg/kg, which can be increased gradually by 1 mg/kg increments until desired response, not to exceed 6 mg/kg. Child weighs 48 lb. On hand is 20 mg/ml.

---

*Calculate kg to nearest tenth. Refer to p. 24 for rounding instructions. For amounts of less than 1 ml, round to nearest hundredth. For amounts of more than 1 ml, round to nearest tenth.

3. Ordered: dactinomycin (actinomycin D, ACT) 0.20 mg IV. Safe pediatric dosage is 15 µg/kg/day. Child weighs 35 lb. On hand is a vial of 0.5 mg/ml.*

4. Ordered: digoxin injection 0.7 mg IV. Safe pediatric dosage for infants to 2 years is 0.03 to 0.05 mg/kg of body weight/24 hr. Baby weighs 26 lb. On hand is 0.1 mg/ml pediatric injection.

5. Ordered: cephapirin sodium (Cefadyl) 0.25 g IV q6h. Safe pediatric dosage for infants is 40 to 80 mg/kg of body weight/24 hr in 4 equally divided doses. Baby weighs 35 lb. On hand is 1 g which must be diluted in 10 ml of sterile water before further dilution.

*When there is only one recommended dose, the medication may be given if it is not an overdose.

Foster, Darryl   Rm 501
Age: 37   Dr. Donalds
91-624-35-3

MEDICATION ADMINISTRATION RECORD

DATE	DRUG DOSE ROUTE		DATE DC	TIME SCHEDULE	DATE 2/8			DATE 2/9			DATE 2/10		
					11-7	7-3	3-11	11-7	7-3	3-11	11-7	7-3	3-11
2/8	Prednisone	IM IV (PO) R SC		qd		0900 C.T.			0900 C.T.			0900 C.T.	
		IM IV PO R SC											
		IM IV PO R SC											
		IM IV PO R SC											
		IM IV PO R SC											
		IM IV PO R SC											
		IM IV PO R SC											
		IM IV PO R SC											
		IM IV PO R SC											
		IM IV PO R SC											
		IM IV PO R SC											
		IM IV PO R SC											
		IM IV PO R SC											
		IM IV PO R SC											
		IM IV PO R SC											
		IM IV PO R SC											
		IM IV PO R SC											
		IM IV PO R SC											
		IM IV PO R SC											

PRN/ONE TIME ONLY ORDERS

DATE	DRUG DOSE ROUTE		DATE DC	TIME SCHEDULE	11-7	7-3	3-11	11-7	7-3	3-11	11-7	7-3	3-11
2/10	Lasix 10 mg	IM IV (PO) R SC		Stat							0530 M.J.		
		IM IV PO R SC											
		IM IV PO R SC											
		IM IV PO R SC											
		IM IV PO R SC											
		IM IV PO R SC											
		IM IV PO R SC											

KEY			Signature	Initials	Signature	Initials	Signature	Initials
ABD - ABDOMEN	**O** - NOT GIVEN	**RA** - RT. ARM	Cathy Tag	C.T.	Cathy Tag	C.T.	Mary Jones	M.J.
LA - LT. ARM	**OD** - RT. EYE	**RT** - RT. THIGH						
LT - LT. THIGH	**OS** - LT. EYE	**RU** - RUQ						

LU - LUQ   **OU** - BOTH EYES

IVPB - IV PIGGYBACK   **SQ** - SUBCUTANEOUS

ALLERGIES
Phenobarbital

■ 145

■ Children's Dosages Test   (Answers on p. 251)

Solve the following problems by using the *mg/kg* rules and make your decisions*:

1. Ordered: tetracycline 200 mg IV bid for a child who weighs 45 lb. Safe range is 10 to 20 mg/kg/day in 2 divided doses. On hand are 250-mg vials of sterile tetracycline hydrochloride that are to be reconstituted initially with 5 ml of sterile water for injection. What is safe dose range for this child? Is the order safe? If so, how many ml will you withdraw from the vial?

2. Ordered: Keflin 250 mg IM q6h for a child who weighs 20 lb, 4 oz. Safe range for children is 80 to 160 mg/kg. What is the safe dose range for this child? Is the order safe? If so, how many ml will you withdraw from the vial? On hand is a 1-g vial that can be reconstituted with 4 ml for IM use.

3. Ordered: furosemide (Lasix) 20 mg po stat for a child. The safe dosage for initial therapy is 2 mg/kg. The child weighed 25 lb today. What is the safe dose for this child's weight? Is the order safe? If so, how many ml will you give? On hand is Lasix Oral Solution 10 mg/ml.

---

*Calculate kg to hundredths.

4. Ordered: furosemide (Lasix) 30 mg IV. Therapeutic range for children is 1 to 6 mg/kg in gradual increments. Child weighs 60 lb. On hand is 20 mg/ml. Calculate the safe dose range for this child's weight and make your decision to give or hold. If the dose is safe, calculate the amount you will give.

5. Ordered: digoxin injection 0.8 mg IV. Safe loading pediatric dose for infants to 2 years is 0.03 to 0.05 mg/kg of body weight q24h. Baby weighs 44 lb. On hand is a vial of 0.5 mg/ml. Calculate the safe dose range and make your decision to give or hold. If the dose is safe, calculate the amount you will give to the nearest hundredth of a ml.

Solve the following problem by using the mg/m^2 rule*:

6. Ordered: Carmustine (BCNU) 200 mg/m^2 IV. Child's BSA in m^2 is 0.9. How many mg will you administer? Available is 3.3 mg/ml. How many ml will you add to the IV infusion?

---

*Refer to BSA mg/m^2 method on p. 132.

Solve the following pediatric problems:

7. Ordered: Mintezol 25 mg/kg of body weight. If the child weighs 20 kg, how many mg will you give? The bottle reads: "Each 5 ml contains 250 mg." How many ml will you give?

8. Ordered: gr iii Liquiprin. Bottle contains 60 mg per 1.25 ml. The dropper measures 2.5 ml. How many ml will you give?

9. On hand is a pediatric oral suspension of Veetids '250' (penicillin-V potassium). The bottle contains 10 g. Directions read: "Add 117 ml water to prepare 200 ml oral solution." Doctor ordered 1 tsp qid × 10 days. How many mg will each teaspoon contain?

10. Average dose of Kantrex (kanamycin sulfate) daily is 750 to 1000 mg. Directions read: "15 mg/kg in divided doses not to exceed 1.5 g in 1 day." The baby weighs 8 lb. How many mg of Kantrex should the baby receive?

CHAPTER 10

Advanced intravenous calculations

Objectives

- Calculate mg/kg, μg/kg per minute and hour.
- Calculate hourly flow rate for titrated intravenous solutions.
- Calculate hourly drug dose for titrated intravenous solutions.
- Estimate infusion rates and drug doses using reduced total drug/total-volume ratios.
- Evaluate infusions for correct flow rate and/or drug dose.
- Calculate time/dose intervals for direct intravenous administration (IV push) with a syringe.

Explanation

Titration is used to administer calculated doses of potent drugs used for dysrhythmias, hypotension, seizures, pain, etc., with dose/flow-rate adjustment based on patient physiologic response to the medication.

The nurse must be able to assess and implement an order for safe and correct dose/flow rate, preferred routes, compatibilities with existing solutions if that tubing will be shared, and evaluate an infusion strength and rate that has been initiated by someone else.*

Titrated drugs may be given by intermittent and continuous intravenous routes. The choice of administration depends on the preferred method cited in the literature for that drug, volume to be administered, equipment and lines available, and condition of the patient.

Small-volume medications may be delivered with a syringe into a vein, a heparin lock, a controlled-volume set such as a buretrol or volutrol container, in secondary IV piggyback equipment, or a port nearest a vein on a primary IV line.†
Large-volume infusions such as magnesium sulfate, which are diluted in 1000 ml, may be given as a primary infusion with an infusion pump.

---

*Flow-rate charts and compatibility charts supplied need to be verified. Some do not cite sources.
†Refer to p. 87 for illustrations of intravenous infusion equipment.

Infusions

Titrated infusions are used to administer drugs such as dopamine, lidocaine, or dobutamine in a continuous infusion in a specified compatible solution, preferably with an infusion pump. If a pump is unavailable, microdrip tubing must be used.* Adjustments to doses are frequent. Control-volume devices such as volutrols or buretrols may be used to limit the amount of titrated infusion available at any one time and must be used for pediatric clients (Fig. 6).

The most potent medications are administered in micrograms/minute μg/kg/min). To reduce errors in flow-rate calculations,† many of these infusions now have a **total-drug:total-volume** ratio of 1:1, 1:2, 1:3 and 1:4 (i.e., 250 mg/250 ml; 250 mg/500 ml). These ratios simplify the mathematics for drug and flow-rate calculation and reduce errors.

If the patient needs fluid restriction, the physician may order a stronger ratio of drug to solution (2:1, 3:1, or 4:1 drug in solution, e.g., 1 g in 250 ml).

Formula for calculating hourly drug and flow rate for titrated infusions

Total drug (TD):total volume (TV)::hourly drug (HD):hourly volume (HV)
in   (one of these will be x)
Lowest reduced ratio   (one of these will be known)

Steps to solving problem:

1. Calculate recommended drug dose/kg/min (μg/kg/min or mg/kg/min) from literature.
2. Compare with physician order using same terms (μg or mg) and evaluate for safe dose.
3. If order is safe, calculate hourly drug and flow rate using the formula that follows (this may necessitate converting mg/μg/min to mg/μg/hr).‡

   EXAMPLE: Ordered: Give 0.3 mg/min of Intropin (dopamine). On hand is 500 mg dissolved in 500 ml 5% D/W. Literature recommends 2 to 5 μg/kg/min, not to exceed 50 μg/kg/min. Titrate to patient response. The patient weighs 242 lb. What flow rate should be set on the pump?

---

*Rates higher than 60 ml/hr (60 gtts/min) are too awkward to count with the microdrip tubing. Titrated infusions seldom require a high flow rate.

†It is essential that the flow rates be correct. "Catching up" to compensate for incorrect flow rates is dangerous.

‡Use of a calculator is helpful.

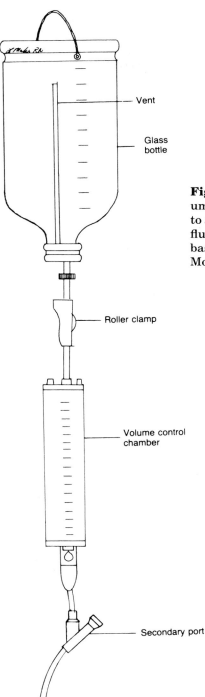

— Vent

Glass
bottle

Fig. 6. Volutrol intravenous administration set. Volume in chamber for pediatric clients should be limited to amount ordered for 1 hour. This protects child from fluid/drug overload. (From Clayton BD, et al: Squire's basic pharmacology for nurses, ed 9, St Louis, 1989, Mosby–Year Book.)

— Roller clamp

Volume control
chamber

Secondary port

Step 1

a. Convert lb to kg (nearest tenth)

1 kg:2.2 lb::x kg:242 lb   PROOF: $1 \times 242 = 242$
2.2x = 242 $2.2 \times 110 = 242$
x = 110 kg

b. Calculate safe-dose range from literature

Know   **Want to know**
2 μg:1 kg::x μg:110 kg   PROOF: $2 \times 110 = 220$
x = 220 μg/min—low therapeutic dose $1 \times 220 = 220$

50 μg:1 kg::x μg:110 kg   PROOF: $50 \times 110 = 5500$
x = 5500 μg/min—high therapeutic dose $1 \times 5500 = 5500$

Safe-dose range is 220 to 5500 μg/min for this patient

Step 2

Compare safe dose range with order.
Safe dose range: 220 to 5500 μg/min.
Ordered: 0.3 mg.
Need to convert mg to μg to compare.

Know   **Want to know**
1000 μg:1 mg::x μg:0.3 mg
x = 1000 × 0.3
x = 300 μg/min ordered
Decision: Give. Order is within safe range.

Step 3

a. Calculate hourly drug dose in mg (same as drug on hand)

Know   **Want to know**   PROOF: $0.3 \times 60 = 18$
0.3 mg:1 min::x mg:60 min $1 \times 18 = 18$
x = 18 mg/hr

b. Calculate hourly rate after reducing the total-drug to total-volume ratio to lowest terms

Total drug:total volume::hourly drug:hourly volume
        500 mg:500 ml::18 mg:x ml   PROOF: $1 \times 18 = 18$
                1:1::18:x $1 \times 18 = 18$
x = 18 ml/hr
Set flow rate on IV machine to 18 ml/hr

Alternative step 3

    If hourly volume is known but hourly drug is not, just place the unknown (x) under hourly drug and fill in the hourly volume ordered in this equation. Then check the answer with the literature for safe range (e.g., the order was for 18 ml/hr or is infusing at 18 ml/hr when you arrive. How much drug is the patient receiving per hour and per minute so that you can compare with literature?)

Use the same formula:
You read the total drug and total volume and hourly volume on the IV set in the room:

Total drug:total volume::hourly drug:hourly volume

500 mg:500 ml::x mg:18 ml

Reduce ratio: 1:1::x:18

    x = 18 mg/hr (1:1 ratio)   PROOF: 18 × 1 = 18

    18 mg:60min:$x$mg:1 min   60 × 0.3 = 18

    60x = 18

    x = 0.3 mg/min

Now you know that the order was followed properly. (You've already checked the literature for a safe range for this patient.)

Worksheet (Answers on p. 252)

1. Change the drug per minute to drug per hour in μg, then mg, for each given weight. Use of a calculator is permissible, or a ratio of given drug × kg:1 minute::x drug:60 minutes. (1000 μg = 1 mg)

	Drug/kg/min	Recommended	μg/hour	mg/hr
a.	5 μg/kg/min	Wt:5 kg	_____	_____
b.	8 μg/kg/min	Wt:20 kg	_____	_____
c.	3 μg/kg/min	Wt:121 lb	_____	_____
d.	4 μg/kg/min	Wt:50 kg	_____	_____
e.	20 μg/kg/min	Wt:60 kg	_____	_____

2. Reduce the total drug:total volume ratio to lowest terms (e.g., 1000:250 = 4: 1)

	Total drug:total volume	Lowest ratio
a.	250 mg:1000 ml	_____
b.	500 mg:500 ml	_____
c.	100 mg:1000 ml	_____
d.	250 mg:500 ml	_____
e.	500 mg:1000 ml	_____

3. Estimate the value of x (hourly volume) after reducing the ratio of total drug to total volume. The ratio of hourly drug to hourly volume will be the same as total drug to total volume.

   Total drug:total volume::hourly drug:hourly volume (ml/hr)
   a. 250 mg:1000 ml::10 mg:x
   b. 500 mg:500 ml::30 mg:x
   c. 100 mg:1000 ml::5 mg:x
   d. 250 mg:500 ml::3 mg:x
   e. 500 mg:250 ml::10 mg:x

4. If you came on duty and evaluated these intravenous solutions and rates in a patient-care setting, you would estimate the hourly drug after reducing the total drug: total volume ratio and then examining the rate set on the infusion pump.

   Estimate the hourly drug (x).

   Total drug:total volume::hourly drug:hourly volume
   a. 250 mg:250 ml::x mg:20 ml
   b. 1000 mg:500 ml::x mg:6 ml
   c. 250 mg:500 ml::x mg:18 ml
   d. 400 mg:1000 ml::x mg:10 ml
   e. 500 mg:250 ml::x mg:18 ml

5. ▪ Change μg to mg by moving the decimal three places to the left.
   ▪ Reduce the total drug:total volume ratio to lowest ratio.
   ▪ Finally, estimate the hourly volume. (Hourly drug must always be calculated in same terms as total drug.)

   Total drug:total volume::hourly drug:hourly volume (ml/hr)
   a. 250 mg:1000 ml::4000 μg (mg):x ml
   b. 500 mg:500 ml::9000 μg (mg):x ml
   c. 1000 mg:500 ml::20,000 μg (mg):x ml
   d. 250 mg:500 ml::15,000 μg (mg):x ml
   e. 400 mg:250 ml::8,000 μg (mg):x ml

Worksheet   (Answers on p. 252)

Tips to ease the work:

Use a calculator to determine weight in kg to nearest tenth. Change μg to mg by moving the decimal three places to the left. Reduce your final total drug:total volume ratio. Label everything.

1. Ordered: dopamine 75 μg/min. Literature states that usual dose is 2 to 5 μg/kg/min. Patient weighs 110 lb. On hand is dopamine 250 mg in 250 D5W.
    ▪ What is safe range/min for this patient's weight?
    ▪ Is order safe?
    ▪ What is hourly drug order in μg? In mg?
    ▪ What is hourly flow rate?

2. Ordered: dobutamine 100 μg/min. On hand is dobutamine 250 mg in 250 ml. The flow rate infusing when you arrive on duty is 5 ml an hour.
    ▪ Is this correct?
    ▪ What is hourly drug order in μg? In mg?
    ▪ What should hourly flow rate be?

3. Ordered: lidocaine 4 mg/minute. On hand is 1 g of lidocaine in 500 ml of 5DW. What flow rate will you set on the infusion pump?

4. Ordered: dobutamine 100 μg/minute for a 150 lb patient. Literature states that usual dose is 2.5 to 10 μg/kg/min. Is this order within the usual dose range? If so, on hand is dobutamine 250 mg in 500 ml 5DW.

5. Ordered: dopamine 500 μg/min for a 72 kg patient. On hand is dopamine 500 mg in 500 ml. The nurse has set the flow rate at 30 ml per hour.
    ▪ Is this correct?
    ▪ The patient response is good. The order is changed to 150 μg/minute. What will you set the flow rate?

Worksheet (Answers on p. 254)

Directions: Use Total drug:total volume::hourly drug:hourly volume (TD:TV::HD:HV) formula. Be sure to reduce TD:TV ratio before doing math. A calculator is helpful for lb to kg and minute to hour conversions.

1. Ordered: 2 mg/min of lidocaine. Available: 1 g lidocaine in 500 ml 5DW. How many mg/hr are ordered? What will the flow rate be? (Change 1 g to mg)

2. Ordered: nitroglycerin IV 5μg/min. Available: 50 mg in 250 ml. How many μg/hour are ordered? How many ml an hour would you set the flow rate on the pump? (Change μg/hr to mg/hr by moving decimal.)

3. Ordered: dopamine 150 μg/min. Literature recommends 2 to 5 μg/kg/min for initial treatment. The patient weighs 110 pounds. What is safe-dose range for this patient? Is the order within the safe range?

   Available is dopamine 250 mg in 250 ml. If safe, what rate would you set on the pump? Follow the sequence: wt in kg; safe-dose range; compare with order; then calculate hourly drug order in μg and mg; calculate hourly flow rate.*

---

*Change μg to mg by moving decimal in μg three places to left.

4. Ordered: dobutamine 5 μg/kg/min. Your patient weighs 80 kg. The nurse has set up the infusion pump with 250 mg dobutamine in 500 ml 5DW at 24 ml/hr. Calculate hourly drug order; change to mg, then calculate ordered ml/hr and compare with current rate. Does the flow rate need changing? If so, what rate will you set?

5. Ordered: nitroprusside sodium 0.25 mg/min for a patient weighing 154 lb. Literature states the safe range is 0.5 μg/kg/min, not to exceed 10 μg/kg/min. What is the safe-dose range? Is the order safe? How much drug per hour is ordered? Available is 50 mg in 250 ml D5W. What would the flow rate be?

10D **Worksheet** (Answers on p. 256)

1. Ordered: magnesium sulfate 2 g/hr IV. You have magnesium sulfate 40 g/1000 ml 5/DNs on an infusion pump.
   - Reduce the ratio of total drug to total volume
   - How many ml/hr will deliver 2 g/hr?
   (Use total drug:total volume:hourly drug:hourly volume formula)

2. Ordered: Pitocin 100 ml/hr IV. You have 1000 ml RLS with 10 U of Pitocin. Literature states maximum dose rarely exceeds 20 mU/min (1000 mU = 1 unit).
   - What is the lowest reduced ratio of total drug to total volume?
   - How much drug per hour in units is safe maximum dose?
   - How much drug per hour is ordered? Is order safe?

3. Ordered: Pitocin 2 mU/min IV. You have 1000 ml of N/S with 20 U of Pitocin.
   - How many mU an hour will be infused?*
   - How many U/hr will be infused?†
   - What is the lowest reduced ratio of total drug to total volume?
   - How many ml an hour will be infused?

4. Ordered: magnesium sulfate 25 ml/hr. Call doctor when 4 g have been infused. You have 500 ml D5W with 20 g of magnesium sulfate on IMED pump.
   - What is lowest reduced ratio of total drug to total volume?
   - How many g/hr will infuse?
   - How long will it take for the 4 g to be infused?

5. Infusing: magnesium sulfate 25 ml/hr. In the room is 250 ml 5D/W with 40 g magnesium sulfate on an infusion pump. Ordered is magnesium sulfate 2 g/hr.
   - What is lowest reduced ratio of total drug to total volume?
   - Is the current flow rate correct? If not, how many ml/hr are ordered?

---

*You may wish to use a calculator and multiply minute dose by 60 to obtain hourly dose.
†Moving the decimal place in mU 3 places to the left will give the equivalent U (1000 mU = 1 u).

Worksheet   (Answers on p. 258)

1. Ordered: aminophylline 50 ml/hr. You have 250 mg of aminophylline in 1000 ml of D5W on an infusion pump. Literature states that safe maintenance range is 0.1 to 0.5 mg/kg/hr for aminophylline.
    - What is the safe-dose range for a patient who weighs 60 kg?
    - What is the lowest reduced ratio of total drug to total volume?
    - How many mg/hr will the patient receive?
    - Is the order safe?

2. Ordered: aminophylline 45 mg/hr. Pharmacy has sent aminophylline 500 mg dissolved in 1000 ml D5W. Literature states 0.5 mg/kg/hr to 0.7 mg/kg/hr for first 12 hours is safe range.
    - What is the safe-dose range for a patient who weighs 80 kg?
    - Is this order safe?
    - What is the lowest reduced ratio of total drug to total volume?
    - If safe, how many ml/hr would you infuse?

3. Ordered: aminophylline 50 ml/hr. You have aminophylline 250 mg in 500 ml of D5W. The recommended maintenance dose is 0.1 to 0.5 mg/kg/hr. The patient weighs 70 kg.
    - What is the safe-dose range for this patient?
    - What is the lowest reduced ratio of total drug to total volume?
    - How many mg of aminophylline will the patient receive per hour?
    - Is the order safe?

4. Ordered: aminophylline 20 mg/hour. You have aminophylline 250 mg in 500 ml D5W. The patient weighs 50 kg. The maximun dose for maintenance is 0.5 mg/kg/hr.
    - What is the maximum safe dose for this patient?
    - Is the order safe?
    - What is the lowest reduced ratio of total drug to total volume?
    - How many ml an hour will the patient receive?

5. Ordered: aminophylline 15 mg/hour. You arrive on duty and your patient's IV is set at 50 ml/hour on an infusion pump. The IV is labelled aminophylline 500 mg in 1000 ml D5W. Your patient weighs 154 pounds and the literature states that the safe range is 0.1 to 0.5 mg/kg/hr.
    - What is the safe range in mg/hr for this patient?
    - Is the order safe?
    - Is the existing flow rate correct for the order?
    - If not, what flow rate would you set?

Direct intravenous administration

Direct intravenous administration (IV push) is used to administer a small amount of diluted or undiluted medication for an acute problem into a vein via a syringe, a heparin lock, a buretrol (or volutrol), or a small, secondary piggyback container. Sometimes it is injected into a port nearest the vein of an existing continuous IV.

In some settings, the nurse may have the option of administering the bolus medication in a volutrol or buretrol or a special 50 ml or 100 ml plastic piggyback container. This may be a desirable option if the medication is to be given over a long period of time, such as 30 to 60 minutes, and if the amount of fluid is great enough to be monitored in the equipment.

Medications that require only a brief administration time or that may be used in an urgent situation, such as dilantin, meperidine, valium, or furesomide, can be administered intravenously by the nurse using a syringe and injecting a diluted or undiluted medication over a period that may vary from as fast as you can inject to several minutes as the literature specifies.

Because these medications are powerful and act rapidly, it is crucial that the literature be consulted for safe-dose limits, rates of flow, dilutions, compatible solutions and routes (IVPB or IV push) and that the patient response be monitored frequently.

Formula for timing IV-push medications

Total volume:total minutes::x volume:1 minute

EXAMPLE: Ordered is furosemide (Lasix) undiluted 40 mg IV-push at 20 mg/min. On hand are 10 mg/1 ml injectable. You plan to begin administration at 16:00. For safe administration it is wise to prepare a brief written schedule that includes start time and some "markers," or "checkpoints," for timing and smooth administration of the injection.

- What is total volume in the syringe you prepare?
- What are logical increments of time and volume as markers for this volume and time period (per minute and each 0.1 ml with small amounts)?
- How many ml will you inject each minute or part of a minute (in seconds)?

Steps to solving problem:

1. Calculate total volume in ml needed for dose ordered.
2. Calculate desired increments using ratio and proportion for volume and minutes in formula (ml and minutes are the "necessary ingredients" for this ratio). Your x may be the volume for each minute or the time for each 0.1 ml.

Determine your start time and write out a schedule of your "markers" (increments of time) and cumulative amount to be infused. Write this before beginning to inject and have it in front of you to avoid errors caused by distraction.

Step 1

Calculate total volume

Have   **Want to know**

10 mg:1 ml::40 mg:x ml

$10x = 40$

$x = 4$ ml total volume for syringe

PROOF: $10 \times 4 = 40$

$1 \times 40 = 40$

Step 2

Calculate volume per minute and parts of a minute

Total volume:total time::x volume:1 minute

(TV)   (TT)

4 ml: 2 min:: x ml:1 minute

PROOF: $4 \times 1 = 4$

$2 \times 2 = 4$

$2x = 4$

$x = 2$ ml/min

Know   **Want to know**

2 ml:60 sec::x ml:15 seconds

$60x = 30$

$x = 0.5$ ml q 15 sec

PROOF: $2 \times 15 = 30$

$60 \times 0.5 = 30$

Schedule: Inject 0.5 ml q 15 sec

1 ml q 30 sec

Start time: 1600:00   4 ml in syringe

1600:30   3 ml remaining

1601:00   2.0 remaining

1601:30   1 ml remaining

1602:00   0 remaining

Worksheet   (Answers on p. 261)

IV push medication schedules

See p. 162-163 for explanation and example.

1. Ordered: 10% calcium chloride (20 ml) over 10 minutes. How many ml/min and ½ min will you inject? Monitor VS and watch the ECG for arrhthymias during the injection.

2. Ordered: Digoxin 1 mg IV. Literature specifies a minimum of 5 minutes for rate of administration. Doctor orders it to be given over 10 minutes. Available: 250 μg/ml. How many total ml will you inject? How many ml/min will you inject? How many ml will you inject every 15 seconds?

3. Ordered: phenytoin sodium IV loading dose of 900 mg at 50 mg/min. Available: 100 mg/ml. How many ml will you inject over how many total minutes? How many ml/min and ½ min will you inject?

4. Ordered: furosemide 20 mg IV over 10 minutes. Available: 10 mg/ml. How many ml will you inject per minute? (Give answer in tenths.)

5. Ordered: meperidine HCl 10 mg IV. Literature states to administer a single dose over 5 minutes. Must be diluted to at least 5 ml of sterile water or normal saline for injection. Available: 50 mg/ml. How many ml will you inject per minute?

CHAPTER 11

Solutions

Objectives

- Calculate percent of sodium chloride in normal saline solution.
- Calculate percent solution problem using ratio and proportion method.*

Explanation

A solution consists of two parts: the solvent (usually water) and the solute (a solid, liquid, or gas) dissolved in the solvent. Solution problems are percent problems. Remember that *percentage* means hundred*ths*. A percent number is a fraction whose top number is stated and bottom number is understood to be 100. 20% is the same as $^{20}/_{100}$. To make a ratio out of a fraction, put the numerator on the left and the denominator on the right. The fraction $^{20}/_{100}$ is the same as the ratio 20:100.

One ml (or cc) of water weighs 1 g. Therefore g and ml (or cc) can be used interchangeably. If the solute (part being dissolved) is a liquid, then ml (or cc) can be used. (The use of ml is preferred over cc, because cc is properly used with gases. Nevertheless, cc is occasionally used in this text.) If the solute is a solid such as NaCl (salt) or tablets, then the g symbol is used.

Normal saline (isotonic sodium chloride) is 0.9%. As a ratio it is *always* written 0.9:100. Half-strength NaCl is 0.45%. As a ratio, it is *always* written 0.45:100.

RULE:	Set up a ratio and proportion with what you *have* on hand on the *left* and what you *want* to make on the *right*.

EXAMPLE: Make up 250 ml of a 20% acetic acid solution.

Have   **Want**

Step 1: 20 ml acetic acid:100 ml water::x ml acetic acid:250 ml water

$100x = 5000$ PROOF: $100 \times 50 = 5000$

$x = 50$ ml acetic acid for a 20% solution $20 \times 250 = 5000$

---

*Few solutions are prepared by nurses.   ■ **165**

When working with liquids such as acetic acid, you must *subtract* the amount of *full-strength* acetic acid needed (in this problem it is 50 ml) from the total amount of solution ordered to determine how much water to add. When you have figured out how much solvent to use, pour exact amount into the container first, then fill to the total amount of solution ordered.

Step 2: Use 50 ml of full-strength acetic acid. The total amount of solution ordered was 250 ml.

> 250 ml ordered
> −50 ml full-strength acetic acid
> ─────────
> 200 ml water added to 50 ml of 20% acetic acid = 250 ml
>   of 20% solution

NOTE: The ratio and proportion setup works when a solution is prepared from a *full-strength* solid or liquid such as salt or 100% solutions.

RULE: If the solution you are to use for the preparation of the desired solution is a ratio, just use the ratio for the *have* side or *left* side of the equation.

EXAMPLE: Make up 1 pint of a 1:1000 Zephiran chloride solution.

Have   **Want**

Step 1: 1 g:1000 ml::x g:500 ml
1000x = 500
x = 0.5 g

Step 2: You will measure ½ g or ml of 1:1000 Zephiran chloride solution and pour it into 499.5 ml of water = 500 ml of 1:1000 solution.

Worksheet (Answers on p. 262)

1. Make up 500 ml of normal saline solution. How many g of salt will you use? How many tsp is this?

2. Make up 200 ml of normal saline. Irrigate wound tid with 60 ml normal saline solution. How many g of salt will you add?

3. Ordered: 300 ml of a 5% acetic acid solution. How much full-strength acetic acid and how much water will you use?

4. Ordered: 250 ml of a 10% acetic acid solution. How much full-strength acetic acid and how much water will you use?

5. Ordered: 150 ml of normal saline solution for a mouthwash. How much salt will you use? How can this problem be simplified?

6. Make up 200 ml of a 10% solution of acetic acid from full-strength liquid. How many ml of acetic acid will you use?

7. Prepare NS solution (0.9%) as an enema. You will use _____ tsp of table salt in 1000 ml of H_2O.

8. Prepare an NS throat irrigation. You will mix _____ tsp of salt with 500 ml H_2O.

9. You are to give 1½% vinegar douche. The douche bag holds 1 qt. You will add _____ tsp of vinegar to 1 qt of H_2O.

10. Prepare 500 ml of a 40% betadine solution using NS.

■ Solutions Test   (Answers on p. 264)

1. Prepare 4 L of a 1:500 ml solution of Lysol. How many ml of Lysol will you need?

2. Prepare 250 ml of a 50% solution of betadine and ½ NS.

3. Prepare 1 L of a 1:750 solution of potassium permanganate. How many g of $KMnO_4$ will you need?

4. Prepare 1 pt of a 1:750 solution of potassium permanganate. Tablets of $KMnO_4$ containing gr 1 each are in stock. How many grains or tablets will you use? Is this a one-step or a two-step problem?

5. Prepare 300 ml of a 30% peroxide solution using 0.9% NS.

Comprehensive examination (Answers on p. 265)

Show work, label answers, and prove.

1. Ordered: elixir of phenobarbital 0.5 g po ac tid. The label reads elixir of phenobarbital 250 mg/ml. How many ml for each dose? How many per day?

2. Ordered: quinidine 200 mg IM. On hand is a vial labeled quinidine 0.1 g/3 ml. How many ml will you give?

3. Ordered: 500 mg of Diuril. On hand are 0.25 g tablets. How many tablets will you give?

4. You are to give atropine 0.3 mg. On hand is a vial labeled 0.4 mg in 0.5 cc. How many ml will you give?

5. You are to give 200,000 units of penicillin. On hand is a multiple-dose vial labeled 1,000,000 U in 10 cc. How many ml will you give?

6. A patient is to receive 500 ml of NS intravenously in 8 hours. How many ml/hr should the patient receive?

7. The above as an IV dose should be infused at _____ gtt/min. Drop factor is 15.

8. The patient is to receive 1000 ml of D5W in 8 hr. How many ml/hr will that be?

9. An IV fluid is being infused at a rate of 100 ml/hr. This should run at _____ gtt/min. Drop factor is 10 gtt/ml.

10. Ordered: penicillin 300,000 units. On hand is a penicillin 5-ml vial stating: "Add 5 ml sterile H$_2$O to make penicillin 600,000 U/2 ml." How many ml will you give?

11. You are to give penicillin 1.3 million units stat. On hand is a vial labeled 10,000,000 units in 10 ml. You will give _____ ml.

12. Ordered: penicillin 600,000 units IM q8h. Available: penicillin 2,000,000 units per 5 ml. You will give _____ ml every 8 hours.

13. Ordered: codeine 10 mg. On hand is 15 mg per ml. How many ml will you give?

14. On hand: codeine (tablets) 0.03 g po. Ordered: 60 mg. How many tablets will you give?

15. Ordered: digoxin 0.125 mg. On hand is an ampule labeled digoxin 0.25 mg/ml. How many ml will you give?

16. Ordered: an IV piggyback of 50 ml in 30 minutes on an infusion pump. At how many ml an hour will you set the rate?

17. Ordered: Dilantin 25 mg tid for a child weighing 33 lb today. Safe dose is 5 mg/kg/day. Is the order safe?

18. Ordered: heparin sodium 5000 U stat. On hand you have a vial labeled heparin sodium 20,000 U per ml. How many ml will you give (nearest hundredth)?

19. Ordered: 75 mg meperidine and Vistaril 25 mg on call to the OR. Have: Demerol 100 mg/ml in a prefilled tube and a 2 ml vial of Vistaril containing 100 mg. How many total ml will you prepare? (Round to nearest tenth.)

20. Ordered: potassium chloride 40 mEq po. On hand you have 20 mEq/15 po. How many ml will you prepare?

21. Ordered: an IV piggyback of 100 ml to infuse in 40 minutes. Drop factor is 10. How many gtts/min will you infuse?

22. Doctor ordered aminophylline suppository 0.5 g. On hand you have aminophylline suppository gr viiss̄. How many will you give?

23. Make up 500 ml of a 20% acetic acid solution. How many ml of acetic acid will you need?

24. Doctor ordered ℥ s̄s̄ of milk of magnesia. How many ml will you give? How many teaspoons is this?

25. Ordered: thyroid tablets 200 mg daily AM. On hand are scored tablets labeled thyroid 0.1 g. How many tablets or what part of a tablet will you give?

26. Your weight is 55 kg. This is equivalent to how many pounds? (Estimate first.)

27. Ordered: prednisone 20 mg for a child with a BSA of 0.5 m². The literature recommends 40 mg/m². Is the order safe? Available is 5 mg/ml. If safe, how much will you give?

28. Ordered: tetracycline 50 mg IV bid for a child who weighs 15 lb, 8 oz. Safe range is 10 to 20 mg/kg/day in two divided doses. On hand are 250-mg vials of sterile tetracycline hydrochloride that are to be reconstituted initially with 5 ml of sterile water for injection. What is the safe dosage range for this child? Is the order safe? If so, how many ml will you withdraw from the vial?

29. Ordered: insulin 8 U/hr IV. Pharmacy has sent 250 ml NS with 50 units regular insulin. How many drops per minute will give you 8 U/hr using microdrip tubing on an infusion pump?

30. Ordered: heparin 500 U/hr IV. Pharmacy has sent 500 ml of D5W with 10,000 units of heparin sodium. How many ml an hour will be needed to infuse 500 U/hr? (Use microdrip.)

Additional formulas for calculation of pediatric doses

Clark's rule

$$\frac{\text{Weight of child in lb}}{150 \text{ lb}} \times \text{Average adult dose} = \text{Child's dose}$$

EXAMPLE: Calculate the dose of atropine sulfate for a child weighing 40 lb. Average adult dose is 0.4 mg/ml.

Weight of child: $\dfrac{40 \text{ lb}}{150 \text{ lb}} \times 0.4$ mg (average adult dose)

$$\frac{40}{150} \times 0.4 = \frac{1.6}{15} = 0.11 \text{ mg}$$

Medication available is atropine sulfate 0.4 mg/ml.

Know   **Want**

0.4 mg:1 ml::0.11 mg:x ml   PROOF: 1 × 0.11 = 0.11

$0.4x = 0.11$ 0.4 × 0.28 = 0.112

$x = 0.28$ ml*

---

*Pediatric volume less than 1 ml should be measured to hundredths in a tuberculin syringe and an appropriate needle size should be selected.

Fried's rule

$$\frac{\text{Age in months}}{150 \text{ months}} \times \text{Average adult dose} = \text{Child's dose}$$

EXAMPLE: Calculate the dose of Valium (diazepam) for an 11-month-old baby if adult dose is 10 mg.

Age in months: $\frac{11}{150} \times 10$ mg (average adult dose)

$$\frac{11}{150} \times 10 = \frac{11\cancel{0}}{15\cancel{0}} = \frac{11}{15} = 0.733$$

Give 0.7 mg of Valium IM.

Available is Valium 10 mg/2 ml ampule. How many ml will you give?

Have	**Want**	
10 mg:2 ml::0.7 mg:x ml		PROOF: $10 \times 0.14 = 1.4$
$10x = 1.4$		$2 \times 0.7 = 1.4$
$x = 0.14$ ml		

Use a tuberculin syringe and measure correct amount.

Young's rule

$$\frac{\text{Age of child in years}}{\text{Age of child} + 12} \times \text{Average adult dose} = \text{Child's dose}$$

EXAMPLE: Calculate the dose of IM Polycillin for a 2 year old if adult dose is 500 mg.

$$\frac{\text{Age}}{\text{Age} + 12} = \frac{2}{2 + 12} \times 500 \text{ mg adult dose} = \frac{2}{14} \times 500 =$$

$$\frac{1}{7} \times \frac{500}{1} = \frac{500}{7} = 71 \text{ mg}$$

Available is Polycillin 500 mg per 2-ml vial. How many ml will you give?

Have	**Want**	
500 mg:2 ml::71 mg:x ml		PROOF: $500 \times 0.28 = 140$
$500x = 142$		$2 \times 71 = 142$
$x = 0.28$ ml		

Answers

General mathematics pretest (p. 1)

1. $6\frac{1}{4}$
2. $5\frac{1}{7}$
3. $\frac{38}{9}$
4. $\frac{19}{2}$
5. 66
6. 45
7. $1\frac{1}{30}$
8. $6\frac{19}{24}$
9. $\frac{13}{28}$
10. $4\frac{7}{8}$
11. $\frac{1}{12}$
12. $\frac{1}{3}$ or $\frac{8}{24}$
13. $\frac{5}{6}$
14. $\frac{18}{40}$ or $\frac{9}{20}$
15. $\frac{1}{50}$
16. $\frac{4}{19}$
17. 0.14
18. 3.016
19. 4.905
20. 28.708
21. 2.96
22. 0.8241
23. 0.0036
24. 1.5
25. 10.055
26. 98.095
27. 0.534
28. 9.125
29. 9.45
30. 73.675
31. $\frac{7}{10}$
32. $\frac{123}{250}$
33. 0.17 and $\frac{17}{100}$
34. 0.125 and 12.5%
35. $\frac{14}{1000}$ and 1.4%

General mathematics

☐ **1A**   (p. 4)

1. 1
2. $3\frac{1}{4}$
3. 3
4. $1\frac{5}{9}$
5. $5\frac{2}{3}$
6. 4
7. $1\frac{3}{4}$
8. $1\frac{7}{8}$
9. 3
10. $6\frac{5}{6}$

☐ **1B**   (p. 5)

1. $\frac{6}{5}$
2. $\frac{5}{4}$
3. $\frac{49}{3}$
4. $\frac{43}{12}$
5. $\frac{68}{5}$
6. $\frac{35}{8}$
7. $\frac{23}{6}$
8. $\frac{21}{8}$
9. $\frac{63}{6}$
10. $\frac{377}{3}$

☐ **1C**   (p. 7)

1.
$$\frac{1}{5}}{\ \ \ +\frac{2}{5}} = \frac{3}{5}$$

   $\frac{1}{5}$
   $+\frac{2}{5}$
   $\frac{3}{5}$

2. $\frac{3}{5} = \frac{9}{15}$
   $+\frac{2}{3} = \frac{10}{15}$
   $\frac{19}{15} = 1\frac{4}{15}$

3. $6\frac{1}{6} = 6\frac{4}{24}$
   $+9\frac{5}{8} = 9\frac{15}{24}$
   $15\frac{19}{24}$

4. $1\frac{3}{8} = 1\frac{15}{40}$
   $+9\frac{9}{10} = 9\frac{36}{40}$
   $10\frac{51}{40} = 11\frac{11}{40}$

5. $2\frac{1}{4} = 2\frac{2}{8}$
   $+3\frac{1}{8} = 3\frac{1}{8}$
   $5\frac{3}{8}$

6. $\frac{1}{8} = \frac{9}{72}$
   $\frac{1}{4} = \frac{18}{72}$
   $+\frac{2}{9} = \frac{16}{72}$
   $\frac{43}{72}$

7. $\frac{7}{9} = \frac{70}{90}$
   $\frac{4}{5} = \frac{72}{90}$
   $+\frac{9}{10} = \frac{81}{90}$
   $\frac{223}{90} = 2\frac{43}{90}$

8. $3\frac{1}{4}$
   $+9\frac{3}{4}$
   $12\frac{4}{4} = 13$

9. $8\frac{2}{5} = 8\frac{4}{10}$
   $14\frac{7}{10} = 14\frac{7}{10}$
   $+9\frac{9}{10} = 9\frac{9}{10}$
   $31\frac{20}{10} = 33$

10. $2\frac{1}{3} = 2\frac{2}{6}$
   $4\frac{1}{6} = 4\frac{1}{6}$
   $6\frac{3}{6} = 6\frac{1}{2}$

1. $\quad 4/5 = 8/10$
    $\quad \underline{-1/2 = 5/10}$
    $\qquad\quad 3/10$

2. $\quad 7^{16}/_{24} = 7^{16}/_{24}$
    $\quad \underline{-3\ ^1/_8\ = 3\ ^3/_{24}}$
    $\qquad\quad 4^{13}/_{24}$

3. $\quad 21\ ^7/_{16} = 20^{23}/_{16}$ $\qquad$ Must borrow from whole number.
    $\quad \underline{-\ \ 7^{12}/_{16} = \ \ 7^{12}/_{16}}$
    $\qquad\qquad\quad 13^{11}/_{16}$

4. $\quad ^{27}/_{32}$
    $\quad \underline{-^{18}/_{32}}$
    $\qquad ^9/_{32}$

5. $\quad 6^3/_{10} = 6^3/_{10}$
    $\quad \underline{-2^1/_5\ = 2^2/_{10}}$
    $\qquad\quad 4^1/_{10}$

6. $\quad 7/_8 = ^{21}/_{24}$
    $\quad \underline{-^2/_3 = ^{16}/_{24}}$
    $\qquad\quad ^5/_{24}$

7. $\quad 3^5/_8$
    $\quad \underline{-1^3/_8}$
    $\qquad 2^2/_8 = 2^1/_4$

8. $\quad 5^3/_7 = 4^{10}/_7$ $\qquad$ Must borrow from whole number.
    $\quad \underline{-1^6/_7 = 1\ ^6/_7}$
    $\qquad\qquad 3\ ^4/_7$

9. $\quad 7\ \ = 6^4/_4$ $\qquad$ Must borrow from whole number.
    $\quad \underline{-1^3/_4 = 1^3/_4}$
    $\qquad\quad 5^1/_4$

10. $\quad 2^7/_8 = 2^7/_8$
    $\quad \underline{-\ \ ^3/_4 = -^6/_8}$
    $\qquad\quad 2^1/_8$

□ **1E** (p. 10)

1. $\frac{1}{3} \times \frac{2}{4} = \frac{2}{12} = \frac{1}{6}$

2. $5\frac{1}{2} \times 3\frac{1}{8} = \frac{11}{2} \times \frac{25}{8} = \frac{275}{16} = 275 \div 16 = 17\frac{3}{16}$

3. $1\frac{3}{4} \times 3\frac{1}{7} = \frac{\overset{1}{\cancel{7}}}{4} \times \frac{22}{\underset{1}{\cancel{7}}} = \frac{22}{4} = 22 \div 4 = 5\frac{1}{2}$

4. $4 \times 3\frac{1}{8} = 4 \times \frac{25}{8} = \frac{100}{8} = 12\frac{1}{2}$

5. $\frac{2}{4} \times 2\frac{1}{6} = \frac{\overset{1}{\cancel{2}}}{4} \times \frac{13}{\underset{3}{\cancel{6}}} = \frac{13}{12} = 1\frac{1}{12}$

6. $\frac{1}{5} \times \frac{1}{3} = \frac{1}{15}$

7. $\frac{3}{4} \times \frac{5}{8} = \frac{15}{32}$

8. $\frac{5}{6} \times 1\frac{9}{16} = \frac{5}{6} \times \frac{25}{16} = \frac{125}{96} = 125 \div 96 = 1\frac{29}{96}$

9. $\frac{5}{100} \times 900 = \frac{5}{\underset{1}{\cancel{100}}} \times \frac{\overset{9}{\cancel{900}}}{1} = 45$

10. $2\frac{1}{10} \times 4\frac{1}{3} = \frac{\overset{7}{\cancel{21}}}{10} \times \frac{13}{\underset{1}{\cancel{3}}} = \frac{91}{10} = 9\frac{1}{10}$

□ **1F** (p. 11)

1. $\frac{2}{5} \div \frac{5}{8} = \frac{2}{5} \times \frac{8}{5} = \frac{16}{25}$

2. $8\frac{3}{4} \div 15 = \frac{\overset{7}{\cancel{35}}}{4} \times \frac{1}{\underset{3}{\cancel{15}}} = \frac{7}{12}$

3. $\frac{3}{4} \div \frac{1}{8} = \frac{3}{\underset{1}{\cancel{4}}} \times \frac{\overset{2}{\cancel{8}}}{1} = 6$

4. $\frac{1}{16} \div \frac{1}{4} = \frac{1}{\underset{4}{\cancel{16}}} \times \frac{\overset{1}{\cancel{4}}}{1} = \frac{1}{4}$

5. $\frac{1}{3} \div \frac{1}{2} = \frac{1}{3} \times \frac{2}{1} = \frac{2}{3}$

6. $\frac{3}{4} \div 6 = \frac{\overset{1}{\cancel{3}}}{4} \times \frac{1}{\underset{2}{\cancel{6}}} = \frac{1}{8}$

7. $2 \div \frac{1}{5} = \frac{2}{1} \times \frac{5}{1} = 10$

8. $3\frac{3}{8} \div 4\frac{1}{2} = \frac{27}{8} \div \frac{9}{2} = \frac{\overset{3}{\cancel{27}}}{\underset{4}{\cancel{8}}} \times \frac{\overset{1}{\cancel{2}}}{\underset{1}{\cancel{9}}} = \frac{3}{4}$

9. $\frac{3}{5} \div \frac{3}{8} = \frac{\overset{1}{\cancel{3}}}{5} \times \frac{8}{\underset{1}{\cancel{3}}} = \frac{8}{5} = 1\frac{3}{5}$

10. $4 \div 2\frac{1}{8} = \frac{4}{1} \times \frac{8}{17} = \frac{32}{17} = 1\frac{15}{17}$

1. ⅓
2. ¹⁄₁₅₀
3. ¹⁄₂₅₀
4. ⅛
5. More
6. Less
7. Less
8. Less
9. More
10. Less

1. Eight hundredths
2. Ninety-two thousandths
3. Seventeen ten-thousandths
4. Three thousand two hundred eighty-seven and four hundred sixty-seven thousandths
5. Six ten-thousandths
6. One hundred and one hundredth
7. 0.36
8. 0.003
9. 0.0008
10. 2.017
11. 0.05
12. 4.1
13. 24.2
14. 15.01
15. 9.0002
16. 3.008
17. 100.018
18. 18.15
19. 0.055
20. 34.1

1.
```
       3.3
  48)158.4
     144
      14 4
      14 4
```

2.
```
          3 3.333
  6.0 )200.0.000
       180
        20 0
        18 0
         2,0 0
         1 80
          2 00
          1 80
            200
            180
```

3.
```
      2.51
  6)15.06
    12
     3 0
     3 0
       6
       6
```

4.
```
        91.264
  0.87 )79.40.000
         78 3
          1 10
           87
           23 0
           17 4
            5 60
            5 22
              380
              348
```

5.
```
        8 60.
  0.78 )670.80.
         624
          46 8
          46 8
```

6.
```
          32.345
  2.43 )78.60.000
         72 9
          5 70
          4 86
           84 0
           72 9
           11 10
            9 72
            1 380
            1 215
```

7.
```
         3.265
  8.2 )26.7.800
       24 6
        2 1 8
        1 6 4
          5 40
          4 92
            480
            410
```

8.
```
          46.107
  5.78 )266.50.000
         231 2
          35 30
          34 68
           62 0
           57 8
            4 200
            4 046
```

9.
```
          1.661
  6.5 )10.8.000
        6 5
        4 30
        3 90
        4 00
        3 90
         100
          65
```

10.
```
       7.653
  10)76.530
     70
      6 5
      6 0
       53
       50
        30
        30
```

1.   0.8
    +0.5
    1.3

2.   3.27
    0.06
    +2.
    5.33

3.   5.01
    +2.999
    8.009

4.   15.6
    0.19
    +200.
    215.79

5.   210.79
    2.
    + 68.4
    281.19

6.   88.6
    576.46
    + 79.
    744.06

7.   6.77
    102.
    + 88.3
    197.07

8.   79.4
    68.44
    + 3.
    150.84

9.   10.56
    +356.4
    366.96

10.   99.7
    +293.23
    392.93 ·

☐ **1K** (p. 19)

1.   3.14
    ×0.002
    0.00628

You do not have to multiply zeros. Count 5 places in from the right, adding zeros where needed.

2.   95.26
    ×1.125
    47630
    19052
    9526
    9526
    107.16750

Count 5 decimal places in from the right.

3.   0.5
    ×100
    50.0

Count 1 decimal place in from the right.

4.   2.14
    ×0.03
    0.0642

Count 4 decimal places in from the right, adding zeros as needed.

5. $\begin{array}{r} 36.8 \\ \times 70.1 \\ \hline 368 \\ 2576 \\ \hline 2579.68 \end{array}$

7. $\begin{array}{r} 90.1 \\ \times 88 \\ \hline 7208 \\ 7208 \\ \hline 7928.8 \end{array}$

9. $\begin{array}{r} 54.5 \\ \times 21 \\ \hline 545 \\ 1090 \\ \hline 1144.5 \end{array}$

6. $\begin{array}{r} 203.7 \\ \times 28 \\ \hline 16296 \\ 4074 \\ \hline 5703.6 \end{array}$

8. $\begin{array}{r} 2.76 \\ \times 0.003 \\ \hline 0.00828 \end{array}$

10. $\begin{array}{r} 200 \\ \times 0.2 \\ \hline 40.0 \end{array}$

□ 1L   (p. 20)

1. $\begin{array}{r} 98.4 \\ -66.50 \\ \hline 31.90 \end{array}$

5. $\begin{array}{r} 266.44 \\ -0.56 \\ \hline 265.88 \end{array}$

9. $\begin{array}{r} 1.723 \\ -0.683 \\ \hline 1.040 \end{array}$

2. $\begin{array}{r} 108.56 \\ -5.40 \\ \hline 103.16 \end{array}$

6. $\begin{array}{r} 7.066 \\ -0.200 \\ \hline 6.866 \end{array}$

10. $\begin{array}{r} 0.8100 \\ -0.6701 \\ \hline 0.1399 \end{array}$

3. $\begin{array}{r} 0.450 \\ -0.367 \\ \hline 0.083 \end{array}$

7. $\begin{array}{r} 34.678 \\ -0.502 \\ \hline 34.176 \end{array}$

4. $\begin{array}{r} 21.78 \\ -19.88 \\ \hline 1.90 \end{array}$

8. $\begin{array}{r} 78.567 \\ -6.77 \\ \hline 71.797 \end{array}$

□ 1M   (p. 22)

1. $\dfrac{4\cancel{0}}{10\cancel{0}} = \dfrac{2}{5}$

5. $1\dfrac{32}{100} = 1^8/_{25}$

8. $\dfrac{2\cancel{0}}{10\cancel{0}} = \dfrac{1}{5}$

2. $\dfrac{8}{10} = \dfrac{4}{5}$

6. $\dfrac{50\cancel{0}}{100\cancel{0}} = \dfrac{1}{2}$

9. $\dfrac{65}{100} = \dfrac{13}{20}$

3. $\dfrac{25\cancel{0}}{100\cancel{0}} = \dfrac{1}{4}$

7. $\dfrac{75\cancel{0}}{100\cancel{0}} = \dfrac{3}{4}$

10. $\dfrac{70\cancel{0}}{100\cancel{0}} = \dfrac{7}{10}$

4. $4\dfrac{08}{100} = 4^2/_{25}$

□ **1N** (p. 23)

1.
```
      0.19
100)19.00
    10 0
     9 00
     9 00
```

2.
```
   1.285
7)9.00
 7
 2 0
 1 4
   60
   56
   40
   35
```

3. $5^9/_{16} = 5 \times 16 + 9 = {}^{89}/_{16}$
```
      5.562½
16)89.000
   80
    9 0
    8 0
    1 00
      96
      40
      32
       8
```

4.
```
   0.2
5)1.0
 1.0
```

5.
```
   0.666
3)2.000
 1 8
   20
   18
   20
   18
```

6.
```
   0.5
2)1.0
 1.0
```

7.
```
      0.083
12)1.000
    96
    40
    36
```

8.
```
   0.75
8)6.00
 5 6
   40
   40
```

9.
```
      0.075
200)15.000
    14 00
     1 000
     1 000
```

10.
```
   2.5
8)20.0
 16
  4 0
  4 0
```

☐ 1O   (p. 25)

Round your answers to the nearest whole number, the nearest tenth, and the nearest hundredth.

		Nearest whole number	Nearest tenth	Nearest hundredth
1.	93.489	93	93.5	93.49
2.	25.430	25	25.4	25.43
3.	38.10	38	38.1	38.10
4.	57.8888	58	57.9	57.89
5.	0.0092	0	0	0.01
6.	3.144	3	3.1	3.14
7.	8.999	9	9.0	9.00
8.	77.788	78	77.8	77.79
9.	12.959	13	13.0	12.96
10.	5.7703	6	5.8	5.77

☐ 1P   (p. 26)

Round your answers to the nearest whole number, the nearest tenth, and the nearest hundredth.

		Nearest whole number	Nearest tenth	Nearest hundredth
1.	$25.3 \times 4.2 =$	106	106.3	106.26
2.	$9.3 \times 2.86 =$	27	26.6	26.60
3.	$4.5 \times 7.57 =$	34	34.1	34.07
4.	$1.3 \times 9.69 =$	13	12.6	12.60
5.	$2.4 \times 5.88 =$	14	14.1	14.11
6.	$8 \div 5 =$	2	1.6	1.60
7.	$4.1 \div 3 =$	1	1.4	1.37
8.	$5 \div 1.2 =$	4	4.2	4.17
9.	$9 \div 2.2 =$	4	4.1	4.09
10.	$10.2 \div 3 =$	3	3.4	3.40

☐ 1Q   (p. 29)

1. Fraction: $\frac{2}{3}$
   Decimal: 0.67

2. Decimal: 0.5
   Percent: 50%

3. Fraction: $\frac{13}{200}$
   Decimal: 0.065

4. Decimal: 0.0833
   Percent: 8.33%

5. Decimal: 0.003
   Percent: 0.3%

6. Fraction: $\frac{1}{10}$
   Percent: 10%

7. Fraction: $\frac{250}{100} = \frac{5}{2}$
   Decimal: 2.5

8. Fraction: $\frac{7}{20}$
   Percent: 35%

9. Decimal: 0.8
   Percent: 80%

10. Fraction: $\frac{78}{100} = \frac{39}{50}$
    Decimal: 0.78

□ **1R** (p. 30)

1.
```
      240
    ×1.14
      960
      240
      240
   273.60
```

2.
```
     1500
      ×.02
     30.00
```

3. $\dfrac{\frac{1}{2}}{100} = \dfrac{1}{2} \div \dfrac{100}{1} = \dfrac{1}{2} \times \dfrac{1}{100} = \dfrac{1}{200} = 200\overline{)1.000}$ .005

```
      9328
      ×.005
    46.640
```
Answer

4. $\dfrac{\frac{1}{3}}{100} = \dfrac{1}{3} \div \dfrac{100}{1} = \dfrac{1}{3} \times \dfrac{1}{100} = \dfrac{1}{300} = 300\overline{)1.000}$ .003
```
      900
      100
```
```
       930
      ×.003
     2.790
```
Answer

5.
```
       50
     ×.28
      400
      100
    14.00
```

6.
```
      200
     ×.09
    18.00
```

7.
```
      400
    ×1.20
     8000
      400
   480.00
```

8.
```
   105.80
     ×.05
   5.2900
```

9.
```
      520
     ×.10
    52.00
```

10.
```
    40.80
     ×.03
   1.2240
```

■ 189

General Mathematics Test (p. 31)

1.	$5\frac{4}{6} = 5\frac{2}{3}$	15.	$\frac{1}{250}$	29.	12.48
2.	$6\frac{6}{7}$	16.	$\frac{2}{13}$	30.	583.00
3.	$\frac{68}{5}$	17.	0.36	31.	$\frac{2}{5}$
4.	$\frac{23}{6}$	18.	2.017	32.	$\frac{57}{200}$
5.	20	19.	8.009	33.	0.43 and $\frac{43}{100}$
6.	40	20.	60.97	34.	0.10 and 10%
7.	$\frac{19}{36}$	21.	3.824	35.	$\frac{29}{1000}$ and 2.9%
8.	$10\frac{7}{8}$	22.	0.1562	36.	8.9
9.	$\frac{5}{24}$	23.	0.000010	37.	1.35
10.	1	24.	3.5	38.	5
11.	$\frac{1}{15}$	25.	3.300	39.	70
12.	$\frac{10}{48} = \frac{5}{24}$	26.	91.264	40.	0.07
13.	$\frac{24}{4} = 6$	27.	1.1875		
14.	$\frac{3}{4}$	28.	8.0625		

Ratio and proportion

☐ 2A (p. 33)

1.	$\frac{2}{4} = \frac{1}{2}$	5.	$\frac{43}{86} = \frac{1}{2}$	8.	$\frac{1}{5}$
2.	$\frac{4}{6} = \frac{2}{3}$	6.	$\frac{2}{13}$	9.	$\frac{1}{150}$
3.	$\frac{2}{500} = \frac{1}{250}$	7.	$\frac{7}{49} = \frac{1}{7}$	10.	$\frac{4}{100} = \frac{1}{25}$
4.	$\frac{6}{1000} = \frac{3}{500}$				

☐ 2B (p. 35)

1. $\frac{1}{2}:x::1:8$
    $1x = \frac{1}{2} \times 8$
    $x = \frac{1}{2} \times \frac{8}{1} = 4$
    $x = 4$

    PROOF: $4 \times 1 = 4$
    $\frac{1}{2} \times 8 = 4$

2. $9:x::5:300$
    $5x = 9 \times 300$
    $5x = 2700$

    $\dfrac{\cancel{5}x}{\cancel{5}} = \dfrac{2700}{5} = 2700 \div 5 = 540$

    $x = 540$

    PROOF: $540 \times 5 = 2700$
    $9 \times 300 = 2700$

3. $\frac{1}{1000}:\frac{1}{100}::x:60$

$\frac{1}{100}x = \frac{1}{1000} \times 60$

$$\frac{1}{100x} = \frac{1}{1000} \times \frac{60}{1} = \frac{1}{50} \times \frac{3}{1} = \frac{3}{50}$$

$$\frac{\frac{1}{100}x}{\frac{1}{100}} = \frac{\frac{3}{50}}{\frac{1}{100}} = \frac{3}{50} \div \frac{1}{100} = \frac{3}{50} \times \frac{100}{1} = 6$$

$x = 6$

PROOF: $\frac{1}{1000} \times 60 = \frac{3}{50}$

$\frac{1}{100} \times 6 = \frac{3}{50}$

4. $\frac{1}{4}:500::x:1000$

$500x = \frac{1}{4} \times 1000$

$$500x = \frac{1}{4} \times \frac{1000}{1} = 250$$

$$\frac{500x}{500} = \frac{250}{500} = 250 \div 500 = 0.5$$

$x = 0.5$

PROOF: $500 \times 0.5 = 250$

$\frac{1}{4} \times 1000 = 250$

5. $36:12::\frac{1}{100}:x$

$36x = 12 \times \frac{1}{100}$

$$36x = \frac{12}{1} \times \frac{1}{100} = \frac{3}{25}$$

$$\frac{36x}{36} = \frac{\frac{3}{25}}{36} = \frac{3}{25} \div 36 = \frac{3}{25} \times \frac{1}{36} = \frac{1}{300}$$

$x = \frac{1}{300}$

PROOF: $36 \times \frac{1}{300} = \frac{3}{25}$

$12 \times \frac{1}{100} = \frac{3}{25}$

6. $6:24::0.75:x$

$6x = 24 \times 0.75 = 18$

$6x = 18$

$$\frac{6x}{6} = \frac{18}{6} = 18 \div 6 = 3$$

$x = 3$

PROOF: $24 \times 0.75 = 18$

$6 \times 3 = 18$

7. $x:600::4:120$

$120x = 4 \times 600 = 2400$

$$\frac{120x}{120} = \frac{2400}{120} = 2400 \div 120 = 20$$

$x = 20$

PROOF: $600 \times 4 = 2400$

$20 \times 120 = 2400$

8. $0.7:70::x:1000$
    $70x = 0.7 \times 1000 = 700$

    $$\frac{\cancel{70}x}{\cancel{70}} = \frac{700}{70} = 700 \div 70 = 10$$

    $x = 10$

PROOF: $70 \times 10 = 700$
$0.7 \times 1000 = 700$

9. $9:27::300:x$
    $9x = 27 \times 300 = 8100$

    $$\frac{\cancel{9}x}{\cancel{9}} = \frac{8100}{9} = 8100 \div 9 = 900$$

    $x = 900$

PROOF: $27 \times 300 = 8100$
$9 \times 900 = 8100$

10. $6:12::\frac{1}{4}:x$
    $6x = 12 \times \frac{1}{4} = 3$

    $$\frac{\cancel{6}x}{\cancel{6}} = \frac{3}{6} = 3 \div 6 = 0.5$$

    $x = 0.5$

PROOF: $12 \times \frac{1}{4} = 3$
$6 \times 0.5 = 3$

□ **2C**   (p. 36)

1. $\frac{1}{200}:x::1:800$
    $1x = \frac{1}{200} \times 800$

    $$1x = \frac{1}{200} \times \frac{800}{1} = 4$$

    $$\frac{\cancel{1}x}{\cancel{1}} = \frac{4}{1} = 4 \div 1 = 4$$

    $x = 4$

PROOF: $4 \times 1 = 4$
$\frac{1}{200} \times 800 = 4$

2. $15:30::x:12$
    $30x = 15 \times 12$
    $30x = 180$

    $$\frac{\cancel{30}x}{\cancel{30}} = \frac{180}{30} = 180 \div 30 = 6$$

    $x = 6$

PROOF: $30 \times 6 = 180$
$15 \times 12 = 180$

3. $\frac{1}{1000} : \frac{1}{100} :: x : 30$

$\frac{1}{100}x = \frac{1}{1000} \times 30$

$$\frac{1}{100}x = \frac{1}{1000} \times \frac{30}{1} = \frac{3}{100}$$

$$\frac{\frac{1}{100}x}{\frac{1}{100}} = \frac{\frac{3}{100}}{\frac{1}{100}} = \frac{3}{100} \div \frac{1}{100} = \frac{3}{100} \times \frac{100}{1} = 3$$

$x = 3$

PROOF: $\frac{1}{1000} \times 30 = \frac{3}{100}$

$\frac{1}{100} \times 3 = \frac{3}{100}$

4. $6 : 12 :: 0.25 : x$

$6x = 12 \times 0.25 = 3$

$$\frac{6x}{6} = \frac{3}{6} = 3 \div 6 = 0.5$$

$x = 0.5$

PROOF: $12 \times 0.25 = 3$

$6 \times 0.5 = 3$

5. $300 : 5 :: x : \frac{1}{60}$

$5x = \frac{1}{60} \times 300$

$$5x = \frac{1}{60} \times \frac{300}{1} = 5$$

$$\frac{5x}{5} = \frac{5}{5} = 5 \div 5 = 1$$

$x = 1$

PROOF: $300 \times \frac{1}{60} = 5$

$5 \times 1 = 5$

6. $\frac{1}{150} : \frac{1}{200} :: 2 : x$

$\frac{1}{150}x = \frac{1}{200} \times 2$

$$\frac{1}{150}x = \frac{1}{200} \times \frac{2}{1} = \frac{1}{100}$$

$$\frac{\frac{1}{150}x}{\frac{1}{150}} = \frac{\frac{1}{100}}{\frac{1}{150}} = \frac{1}{100} \div \frac{1}{150} = \frac{1}{100} \times \frac{150}{1} = \frac{3}{2} = 1\frac{1}{2}$$

$x = 1\frac{1}{2}$

PROOF: $\frac{1}{150} \times 1\frac{1}{2} = \frac{1}{100}$

$\frac{1}{200} \times 2 = \frac{1}{100}$

7. $\frac{1}{2} : \frac{1}{6} :: \frac{1}{4} : x$

$\frac{1}{2}x = \frac{1}{6} \times \frac{1}{4} = \frac{1}{24}$

$$\frac{\frac{1}{2}x}{\frac{1}{2}} = \frac{\frac{1}{24}}{\frac{1}{2}} = \frac{1}{24} \div \frac{1}{2} = \frac{1}{24} \times \frac{2}{1} = \frac{1}{12}$$

$x = \frac{1}{12}$

PROOF: $\frac{1}{2} \times \frac{1}{12} = \frac{1}{24}$

$\frac{1}{6} \times \frac{1}{4} = \frac{1}{24}$

8. $7.5:12::x:28$
   $12x = 7.5 \times 28 = 210$

   $\dfrac{\cancel{12}x}{\cancel{12}} = \dfrac{210}{12} = 210 \div 12 = 17.5$

   $x = 17.5$

PROOF: $7.5 \times 28 = 210$
$12 \times 17.5 = 210$

9. $15:x::1.5:10$
   $1.5x = 15 \times 10 = 150$

   $\dfrac{\cancel{1.5}x}{\cancel{1.5}} = \dfrac{150}{1.5} = 150 \div 1.5 = 100$

   $x = 100$

PROOF: $15 \times 10 = 150$
$100 \times 1.5 = 150$

10. $10:x::0.4:12$
    $0.4x = 10 \times 12 = 120$

    $\dfrac{\cancel{.4}x}{\cancel{.4}} = \dfrac{120}{.4} = 120 \div .4 = 300$

    $x = 300$

PROOF: $10 \times 12 = 120$
$300 \times 0.4 = 120$

☐ **2D** (p. 38)

1. **Have**   **Want to know**
   Scoops:Cups::Scoops:Cups
   $4:6::x:18$
   $6x = 72$

   $\dfrac{\cancel{6}x}{\cancel{6}} = \dfrac{72}{6} = 12$

   $x = 12$ scoops of cocoa

PROOF: $4:6::12:18$
$6 \times 12 = 72$
$4 \times 18 = 72$

REMEMBER: Scoops:Cups::Scoops:Cups
Apples:Bananas::Apples:Bananas
Miles:Gallons::Miles:Gallons

You want x to stand alone. To get x to stand alone, divide by 6. Whatever you do on one side of an equation, you must do on the other.

Obtain proof by putting your answer back into the equation in place of x. Multiply the two inside numbers, and they should equal the two outside numbers.

2. **Have**　　　　**Want to know**
Scoops:Cups::Scoops:Cups
$7:8::x:40$
$8x = 40 \times 7 = 280$

$$\frac{\cancel{8}x}{\cancel{8}} = \frac{280}{8} = 35$$

$x = 35$ scoops

3. **Have**　　　　**Want to know**
Bananas:Apples::Bananas:Apples
$6:9::x:72$
$9x = 6 \times 72 = 432$

$$\frac{\cancel{9}x}{\cancel{9}} = \frac{432}{9} = 48$$

$x = 48$ bananas

4. **Have**　　　　**Want to know**
300 mg:1 tab.::450 mg:x tab.
$300x = 450$

$$\frac{\cancel{300}x}{\cancel{300}} = \frac{450}{300} = 1.5$$

$x = 1.5$ tab.

Always label your answer.

5. **Have**　　　　**Want to know**
Bushes:Trees::Bushes:Trees
$8:2::x:36$
$2x = 8 \times 36 = 288$

$$\frac{\cancel{2}x}{\cancel{2}} = \frac{288}{2} = 144$$

$x = 144$ bushes

6. **Have**　　　**Want to know**
Cups:Day::Cups:Day
$4:1::84:x$
$4x = 84$

$$\frac{\cancel{4}x}{\cancel{4}} = \frac{84}{4} = 21$$

$x = 21$ days

7. **Have**   **Want to know**

   Cups:Loaves::Cups:Loaves
   $4:3::24:x$
   $4x = 72$

   $$\frac{\cancel{4}x}{\cancel{4}} = \frac{72}{4} = 18$$

   $x = 18$ loaves

                                                    PROOF: $4:3::24:18$
                                                    $4 \times 18 = 72$
                                                    $3 \times 24 = 72$

8. **Have**   **Want to know**

   3 soda:½ fruit juice::x soda:2 fruit juice
   $\frac{1}{2}x = 3 \times 2$

   $$\frac{\frac{1}{2}x}{\frac{1}{2}} = \frac{6}{\frac{1}{2}} = 12$$

   $x = 12$ cups soda

                                                    PROOF: $3:\frac{1}{2}::12:2$
                                                    $3 \times 2 = 6$
                                                    $\frac{1}{2} \times 12 = 6$

9. **Have**   **Want to know**

   4 tbsp sugar:1 glass::x tbsp sugar:6 glasses
   $x = 6 \times 4 = 24$
   $x = 24$ tbsp sugar

                                                    PROOF: $4:1::24:6$
                                                    $4 \times 6 = 24$
                                                    $1 \times 24 = 24$

10. **Have**   **Want to know**

   4 capsules:1 day::x capsules:14 days
   $x = 4 \times 14 = 56$
   $x = 56$ capsules

                                                    PROOF: $4:1::56:14$
                                                    $4 \times 14 = 56$
                                                    $1 \times 56 = 56$

□ **2E**   (p. 41)

1. **Have**   **Want to know**

   200 envelopes:1 box::4000 envelopes:x boxes
   $200x = 4000$

   $$\frac{\cancel{200}x}{\cancel{200}} = \frac{\cancel{4000}}{\cancel{200}}$$

   $\cancel{x} = 20$ boxes

                                                    PROOF: $200 \times 20 = 4000$
                                                    $1 \times 4000 = 4000$

2. **Have**   **Want to know**

   10 disks:1 package::300 disks:x packages
   $10x = 300$

   $$\frac{\cancel{10}x}{\cancel{10}} = \frac{\cancel{300}}{\cancel{10}} = 30 \text{ packages}$$

                                                    PROOF: $10 \times 30 = 300$
                                                    $1 \times 300 = 300$

3. **Have**

              Want to know

1 computer:18 students::x computers:1280 students

$18x = 1280$

$$\frac{\cancel{18}x}{\cancel{18}} = \frac{1280}{18}$$

$x = 71.1$ or 71 computers

PROOF: $1 \times 1280 = 1280$

$18 \times 71.1 = 1279.8$ or 1280

4. **Have**

              Want to know

3 water:2 apples::24 water:x apples

$3x = 48$

$$\frac{\cancel{3}x}{\cancel{3}} = \frac{48}{3} = 16$$

$x = 16$ apples

PROOF: $3:2::24:16$

$3 \times 16 = 48$

$2 \times 24 = 48$

5. **Have**

              Want to know

6 pens:8 pencils::x pens:72 pencils

$8x = 432$

$$\frac{\cancel{8}x}{\cancel{8}} = \frac{432}{8} = 54$$

$x = 54$ pens

PROOF: $6:8::54:72$

$6 \times 72 = 432$

$8 \times 54 = 432$

6. **Have**

              Want to know

½ tsp salt:3 eggs::x tsp salt:30 eggs

$3x = 30 \times \frac{1}{2}$

$$3x = \frac{30}{1} \times \frac{1}{2} = \frac{30}{2} = 15$$

$$\frac{\cancel{3}x}{\cancel{3}} = \frac{15}{3} = 5$$

$x = 5$ tsp salt

PROOF: $½:3::5:30$

$3 \times 5 = 15$

$½ \times 30 = 15$

7. **Have**

              Want to know

8 cups:7 scoops::24 cups:x scoops

$8x = 7 \times 24$

$$\frac{\cancel{8}x}{\cancel{8}} = \frac{168}{8} = 21$$

$x = 21$ scoops

PROOF: $8:7::24:21$

$8 \times 21 = 168$

$7 \times 24 = 168$

8. **Have**   **Want to know**

    Carnations:Ferns::Carnations:Ferns   PROOF: 5:1::50:10

    $5:1::x:10$ $5 \times 10 = 50$

    $x = 5 \times 10$ $1 \times 50 = 50$

    $x = 50$ carnations

9. **Have**   **Want to know**

    Vinegar:Water::Vinegar:Water   PROOF: 2:1::20:10

    $2:1::x:10$ $2 \times 10 = 20$

    $x = 2 \times 10$ $1 \times 20 = 20$

    $x = 20$ tbsp vinegar

10. **Have**   **Want to know**

    ½ milk:3 C flour::x milk:21 C flour   PROOF: ½ × 21 = 10.5

    $3x = \frac{1}{2} \times 21$ $3 \times 3.5 = 10.5$

$$\frac{\cancel{3}x}{\cancel{3}} = \frac{10.5}{3}$$

    $x = 3.5$ cups milk

□ **2F**   (p. 43)

1. **Have**   **Want to know**

    10 centerpieces:1 carton::120 centerpieces:x cartons   PROOF: $10 \times 12 = 120$

    $10x = 120$ $1 \times 120 = 120$

$$\frac{10x}{10} = \frac{120}{10}$$

    $x = 12$ cartons

2. **Have**   **Want to know**

    4 tsp:1 day::80 tsp:x days   PROOF: $4 \times 20 = 80$

    $4x = 80$ $1 \times 80 = 80$

$$\frac{4x}{4} = \frac{80}{4}$$

    $x = 20$ days

3. **Have**   **Want to know**

    10 diapers:1 day::50 diapers:x days   PROOF: $10 \times 5 = 50$

    $10x = 50$ $1 \times 50 = 50$

$$\frac{10x}{10} = \frac{50}{10}$$

    $x = 5$ days

4. **Have**   **Want to know**

    3 drops:2 eggs::x drops:12 eggs   PROOF: $3 \times 12 = 36$

    $2x = 36$ $2 \times 18 = 36$

    $x = 18$ drops

5. **Have**   **Want to know**

    1.5 bathrooms:1 aptmt::x bathrooms:75 apartments   PROOF: $1.5 \times 75 = 112.5$

    $x = 75 \times 1.5$ or 112.5 bathrooms $1 \times 112.5 = 112.5$

    Have   **Want to know**

    3 towels:1 bathroom::x towels:112.5 bathrooms   PROOF: $3 \times 112.5 = 337.5$ or 338

    $x = 3 \times 112.5$ or 337.5 towels (338) $1 \times 337.5 = 337.5$ or 338

☐ **2G**   (p. 44)

1. **Have**   **Want to know**

    35 books:1 shelf::280 books:x shelves   PROOF: $35 \times 8 = 280$

    $35x = 280$ $1 \times 280 = 280$

$$\frac{\cancel{35}x}{\cancel{35}} = \frac{280}{35}$$

    $x = 8$ shelves

2. **Have**   **Want to know**

    2 tbsp:½ cup::x tbsp:6 cups   PROOF: $2 \times 6 = 12$

    $½x = 6 \times 2$ or 12 $½ \times 24 = 12$

$$\frac{½x}{\cancel{½}} = \frac{12}{½}$$

    $x = 24$ tbsp

3. **Have**   **Want to know**

    60 lines:1 page::1800 lines:x pages   PROOF: $60 \times 30 = 1800$

    $60x = 1800$ $1 \times 1800 = 1800$

$$\frac{\cancel{60}x}{\cancel{60}} = \frac{1800}{60}$$

    $x = 30$ pages

4. **Have**   **Want to know**

    1 change:2500 miles::x changes:100,000 miles   PROOF: $2500 \times 40 = 100000$

    $2500x = 100,000$ $1 \times 100,000 = 100000$

$$\frac{\cancel{2500}x}{\cancel{2500}} = \frac{100,000}{2500}$$

    $x = 40$ changes

5. **Have** **Want to know**

4 cookies:6 guests::x cookies:54 guests

$6x = 216$

PROOF: $4 \times 54 = 216$

$6 \times 36 = 216$

$$\frac{\cancel{6}x}{\cancel{6}} = \frac{216}{6}$$

$x = 36$ cookies

Ratio and Proportion Test   (p. 45)

1. 540	5. 9000	8. 0.5 or ½
2. 3	6. 10	9. 1000
3. 12	7. 900	10. 8⅓
4. 20		

Metric system

☐ **3A**   (p. 49)

1. 1000 mg	8. 100 mg	15. 15 g
2. 2000 mg	9. 1100 mg	16. 0.010 g
3. 1500 mg	10. 300 mg	17. 0.100 g
4. 500 mg	11. 0.025 g	18. 0.0005 g
5. 500 mg	12. 0.005 g	19. 0.0075 g
6. 250 mg	13. 3 g	20. 0.02015 g
7. 50 mg	14. 1.5 g	

☐ **3B**   (p. 51)

1. **Know** **Want to know**

1000 mg:1 g::25 mg:x g

PROOF: $1000 \times 0.025 = 25$

$1 \times 25 = 25$

$$\frac{\cancel{1000}x}{\cancel{1000}} = \frac{25}{1000} = 25 \div 1000$$

$x = 0.025$ g

2. **Know**   **Want to know**

1000 mg:1 g::x mg:0.064 g

$1x = 1000 \times 0.064$

$x = 64$ mg

PROOF: $1 \times 64 = 64$

$1000 \times 0.064 = 64$

3. **Know**   **Want to know**

1000 mg:1 g::4 mg:x g

$1000x = 4$

$$\frac{\cancel{1000}x}{\cancel{1000}} = \frac{4}{1000} = 4 \div 1000$$

$x = 0.004$ g

PROOF: $1000 \times 0.004 = 4$

$1 \times 4 = 4$

4. **Know**   **Want to know**

1000 mg:1 g::x mg:4.6 g

$1x = 1000 \times 4.6$

$x = 4600$ mg

PROOF: $1 \times 4600 = 4600$

$1000 \times 4.6 = 4600$

5. **Know**   **Want to know**

1000 ml:1 L::375 ml:x L

$1000x = 375$

$$\frac{\cancel{1000}x}{\cancel{1000}} = \frac{375}{1000} = 375 \div 1000$$

$x = 0.375$ L

PROOF: $0.375 \times 1000 = 375$

$1 \times 375 = 375$

6. **Know**   **Want to know**

1000 g:1 kg::x g:89 kg

$1x = 89{,}000$

$x = 89{,}000$ g

PROOF: $1 \times 89{,}000 = 89{,}000$

$1000 \times 89 = 89{,}000$

7. **Know**   **Want to know**

1000 μg:1 mg::x μg:45 mg

$x = 1000 \times 45$

$x = 45{,}000$ μg

PROOF: $1000 \times 45 = 45{,}000$

$1 \times 45{,}000 = 45{,}000$

8. **Know**   **Want to know**

1000 mg:1 g::x mg:0.6 g

$1x = 1000 \times 0.6$

$x = 600$ mg

PROOF: $1 \times 600 = 600$

$1000 \times 0.6 = 600$

9. **Know**   **Want to know**

1 kg:2.2 lb::50 kg:x lb

$1x = 50 \times 2.2$

$x = 110$ lb

PROOF: $2.2 \times 50 = 110$

$1 \times 110 = 110$

10. **Know**   **Want to know**

1000 g:2.2 lb::2500 g:x lb

$1000x = 2.2 \times 2500 = 5500$

$x = 5.5$ lb

PROOF: $2.2 \times 2500 = 5500$

$1000 \times 5.5 = 5500$

☐ **3C**   (p. 52)

1. **Have**   **Want to know**

10 mg:1 tablet::5 mg:x tablets

$10x = 5$

$$\frac{\cancel{10}x}{\cancel{10}} = \frac{5}{10}$$

$x = 0.5$ or ½ tablet*

PROOF: $10 \times 0.5 = 5$

$1 \times 5 = 5$

2. **Have**   **Want to know**

0.05 g:1 capsule::0.1 g:x capsules

$0.05x = 0.1$

$$\frac{\cancel{0.05}x}{\cancel{0.05}} = \frac{0.1}{0.05}$$

$x = 2$ capsules

PROOF: $0.05 \times 2 = 0.1$

$1 \times .1 = 1$

3. **Have**   **Want to know**

250 mg:1 capsule::500 mg:x capsules

$250x = 500$

$$\frac{\cancel{250}x}{\cancel{250}} = \frac{500}{250}$$

$x = 2$ capsules

PROOF: $250 \times 2 = 500$

$1 \times 500 = 500$

4. **Have**   **Want to know**

1 g:10 ml::0.25 g:x ml

$x = 10 \times 0.25$ or 2.5 ml

PROOF: $1 \times 2.5 = 2.5$

$10 \times 0.25 = 2.5$

---

*Only break scored tablets in half. If unavailable, call pharmacy.

5. **Have**   **Want to know**

30 mg:1 tablet::15 mg:x tablets

$30x = 15$

$$\frac{\cancel{30}x}{\cancel{30}} = \frac{15}{30}$$

$x = 0.5$ or ½ tablet

PROOF: $30 \times ½ = 15$

        $1 \times 15 = 15$

☐ **3D**   (p. 54)

1. *Step 1*

Know   **Want to know**

1000 mg:1 g::x mg:0.75 g

$1x = 750$

$x = 750$ mg

PROOF: $1000 \times 0.75 = 750$

        $1 \times 750 = 750$

Must change g into mg because that is what is available.

Step 2

Know or have   **Want to know**

250 mg:1 tab.::750 mg:x tab.

$$\frac{\cancel{250}x}{\cancel{250}} = \frac{750}{250} = 750 \div 250$$

$x = 3$ tab.

PROOF: $250 \times 3 = 750$

        $1 \times 750 = 750$

You must give 3 tablets of 250 mg each to give required amount of 750 mg.

2. *Step 1*

Know   **Want to know**

1000 mg:1 g::10 mg:x g

$1000x = 10$

$x = 0.01$ g

PROOF: $1000 \times 0.01 = 10$

        $1 \times 10 = 10$

Step 2

Know or have   **Want to know**

0.005 g:1 tab.::0.01 g:x tab.

$$\frac{\cancel{0.005}x}{\cancel{0.005}} = \frac{0.01}{0.005}$$

$x = 2$ tab. of 0.005 g

PROOF: $1 \times 0.01 = 0.01$

        $0.005 \times 2 = 0.01$

3. *Step 1*

   Know   **Want to know**
   1000 mg:1 g::4 mg:x g
   1000x = 4
   x = 0.004 g

   PROOF: $1 \times 4 = 4$
   $1000 \times 0.004 = 4$

   Step 2

   Know or have   **Want to know**
   0.002 g:1 tab.::0.004 g:x tab.
   0.002x = 0.004
   x = 2 tab.

   PROOF: $1 \times 0.004 = 0.004$
   $0.002 \times 2 = 0.004$

   You will give 2 tablets of 0.002g

4. *Step 1*

   Know   **Want to know**
   1000 mg:1 g::75 mg:x g
   1000x = 75
   x = 0.075 g

   PROOF: $1 \times 75 = 75$
   $1000 \times 0.075 = 75$

   Step 2

   Know or have Want to know
   0.050 g:1 ml::0.075 g:x ml
   0.050x = 0.075
   x = 1.5 ml or 1½ ml

   PROOF: $1 \times 0.075 = 0.075$
   $0.050 \times 1.5 = 0.075$

5. *Step 1*

   Know   **Want to know**
   1000 mg:1 g::x mg:0.075 g
   1x = 75 mg
   x = 75 mg

   PROOF: $1 \times 75 = 75$
   $1000 \times 0.075 = 75$

   Step 2

   Know or have   **Want to know**
   25 mg : 1 ml :: 75 mg:x ml
   25x = 75
   x = 3 ml

   PROOF: $1 \times 75 = 75$
   $25 \times 3 = 75$

6. *Step 1*

   Know   **Want to know**
   1000 mg:1 g::x mg:2 g
   1x = 2000
   x = 2000 mg

   PROOF: $1 \times 2000 = 2000$
   $1000 \times 2 = 2000$

Step 2

Know or have Want to know
500 mg:1 ml::2000 mg:x ml
$500x = 2000$
$x = 4$ ml

PROOF: $1 \times 2000 = 2000$
$500 \times 4 = 2000$

7. *Step 1:*

Know   **Want to know**
1000 mg:1 g::500 mg:x g
$1000x = 500$
$x = 0.5$ g

PROOF: $1 \times 500 = 500$
$1000 \times 0.5 = 500$

Step 2

Know or have Want to know
0.25 g:1 tab.::0.5 g:x tab.
$0.25x = 0.5$
$x = 2$ tab.

PROOF: $1 \times 0.5 = 0.5$
$0.25 \times 2 = 0.5$

8. *Step 1*

Know   **Want to know**
1000 mg:1 g::x mg:0.125 g
$1x = 125$
$x = 125$ mg

PROOF: $1000 \times 0.125 = 125$
$1 \times 125 = 125$

Step 2

Know or have Want to know
50 mg:5 ml::125 mg:x ml
$50x = 625$
$x = 12.5$ ml of Keflin IV

PROOF: $50 \times 12.5 = 625$
$5 \times 125 = 625$

9. *Step 1*

Know   **Want to know**
1000 mg:1 g::x mg:.002 g
$x = 2$ mg

PROOF: $1000 \times .002 = 2$
$2 \times 1 = 2$

Step 2:

Know or have Want to know
1 mg:1 tab.::2 mg:x tab.
$x = 2$ tab.

PROOF: $1 \times 2 = 2$
$2 \times 1 = 2$

10. **Know or have**   **Want to know**

    5 mg : 2 ml :: 2 mg : x ml

    $5x = 4$

    $x = 0.8$ ml

PROOF: $2 \times 2 = 4$

             $5 \times 0.8 = 4$

CHAPTER 3

Metric System Test   (p. 57)

---

1. 0.5 g
2. 0.025 g
3. 5000 μg
4. 200 mg
5. 4000 mg

6. ½ tab. (two-step problem)
7. 3 tab. (one-step problem)
8. 3 tab. (two-step problem)
9. 2 tab.
10. 2 tab.

CHAPTER 4

Apothecary/metric system conversions

☐ **4A**   (p. 62)

REMEMBER: *Have* or *know* goes on the left.

1. **Have**   **Want to know**

    gr ½ : 1 ml :: gr 1 : x ml

$$\frac{\tfrac{1}{2}x}{\tfrac{1}{2}} = \frac{1}{\tfrac{1}{2}} = 1 \div \tfrac{1}{2} = 1 \times 2 = 2$$

    $x = 2$ ml

PROOF: $\tfrac{1}{2} \times 2 = 1$

         $1 \times 1 = 1$

2. **Have**   **Want to know**

    gr 5 : 1 tab. :: gr 15 : x tab.

    $5x = 15$

    $x = 3$ tab.

PROOF: $5 \times 3 = 15$

        $1 \times 15 = 15$

3. **Have**   **Want to know**

    gr ⅛ : 1 ml :: gr ⅙ : x ml

$$\frac{\tfrac{1}{8}x}{\tfrac{1}{8}} = \frac{\tfrac{1}{6}}{\tfrac{1}{8}} = \frac{1}{6} \div \frac{1}{8} = \frac{1}{6} \times \frac{8}{1} = \frac{4}{3} = 1\tfrac{1}{3}$$

    $x = 1\tfrac{1}{3}$ ml

PROOF: $\tfrac{1}{8} \times 1\tfrac{1}{3} = \tfrac{1}{6}$

        $1 \times \tfrac{1}{6} = \tfrac{1}{6}$

$$\text{Answer must be a decimal. Therefore: } 1\tfrac{1}{3} = \tfrac{4}{3} = 3\overline{)4.00} \quad \begin{array}{r} 1.33 = 1.33 \\ \hline \\ \underline{3} \\ 1\,0 \\ \underline{9} \\ 10 \\ \underline{9} \\ 1 \end{array}$$

Give 1.3 ml of morphine sulfate.

4. This is a two-step problem.

   Know   Want to know

   $\bar{3}\,\dot{i}{:}1 \text{ tsp}{::}\bar{3}\,\ddot{ii}{:}x \text{ tsp}$ PROOF: $1 \times 2 = 2$

   $x = 1 \times 2 = 2$ $1 \times 2 = 2$

   $x = 2 \text{ tsp}$

   Know   Want to know

   $1 \text{ tsp}{:}5 \text{ ml}{::}2 \text{ tsp}{:}x \text{ ml}$ PROOF: $1 \times 10 = 10$

   $x = 5 \times 2 = 10$ $5 \times 2 = 10$

   $x = 10 \text{ ml}$

5. What do you know about $\bar{3}$ and ml?

   Know   Want to know

   $30 \text{ ml}{:}1 \text{ oz}{::}x \text{ ml}{:}\tfrac{1}{2} \text{ oz}$ PROOF: $30 \times \tfrac{1}{2} = 15$

   $1x = 30 \times \dfrac{1}{2} = 15$ $1 \times 15 = 15$

   $x = 15 \text{ ml of Maalox}$

   The fact that the bottle contained 8 oz of Maalox has nothing to do with the relationship between ml and 1 oz.

6. Give less than 1 ml.

   Have   Want to know

   $\text{gr } \tfrac{1}{4}{:}1 \text{ ml}{::}\text{gr } \tfrac{1}{6}{:}x \text{ ml}$ PROOF: $\tfrac{1}{4} \times \tfrac{2}{3} = \tfrac{1}{6}$

   $\dfrac{1}{4}x = \dfrac{1}{6}$ $1 \times \tfrac{1}{6} = \tfrac{1}{6}$

   $\dfrac{1}{6} \div \dfrac{1}{4} = \dfrac{1}{6} \times \dfrac{4}{1} = \tfrac{2}{3}$

   $x = \tfrac{2}{3} \text{ ml}$

Answer must be a decimal. $\frac{2}{3} = 3\overline{)2.00}$

$$3\overline{)2.00} \quad .66$$

$$\frac{1\,8}{20}$$

$$\frac{18}{2}$$

Give 0.66 ml of codeine sulfate SC.

7. **Have**   **Want to know**

gr ½:1 capsule::gr 1½:x capsules

½x = 1½

$$\frac{\cancel{½}x}{\cancel{½}} = \frac{3/2}{1/2}$$

$\frac{3}{2} \times \frac{2}{1} = \frac{6}{2} = 3$

Give 3 capsules.

PROOF: ½ × 3 = 1½
            1 × 1½ = 1½

8. This is a two-step problem.

Have   **Want to know**

gr $\frac{1}{150}$:½ ml::gr $\frac{1}{200}$:x ml

$$\frac{1}{150}x = \frac{1}{2} \times \frac{1}{200} = \frac{1}{400}$$

$$\frac{\cancel{1/150}x}{\cancel{1/150}} = \frac{1/400}{1/150} = \frac{1}{400} \times \frac{150}{1} = \frac{3}{8}$$

x = 0.37 ml

PROOF: ½ × $\frac{1}{200}$ = $\frac{1}{400}$
            $\frac{1}{150}$ × $\frac{3}{8}$ = $\frac{1}{400}$

You may either change fraction to decimal or leave it as it is for working out the remainder of the problem.

9. **Have**   **Want to know**

gr 5:1 tab.::gr 15:x tab.

5x = 15

x = 3 tab.

PROOF: 5 × 3 = 15
            1 × 15 = 15

10. **Know**   **Want to know**

    30 ml:℥i::x ml:℥ $\overline{ss}$

    $x = 15$ ml

PROOF: ½ × 30 = 15

            1 × 15 = 15

☐ **4B**   (p. 66)

1. **Know**   **Want to know**

    1.0 g:gr 15::x g:gr 10
    $15x = 10 = 10 \div 15 = 0.66$
    $x = 0.66$g

PROOF: 15 × 0.66 = 9.9 = 10

            1 × 10 = 10

2. **Know**   **Want to know**

    1.0 g:gr 15::0.5 g:gr x
    $1x = 15 \times 0.5 = 7.5$
    $x = $ gr 7.5

PROOF: 15 × 0.5 = 7.5

            1 × 7.5 = 7.5

3. **Know**   **Want to know**

    1.0 g:gr 15::x g:gr 7½
    $15x = 7½$
    $x = 0.5$ g

PROOF: 15 × 0.5 = 7.5

            1 × 7.5 = 7.5

4. **Know**   **Want to know**

    60.0 mg:gr i::x mg:gr ¾
    $1x = 60 \times ¾ = 45$
    $x = 45$ mg

PROOF: 1 × 45 = 45

            60 × ¾ = 45

5. **Know**   **Want to know**

    60 mg:gr 1::x mg:gr ¹⁄₁₅₀

    $1x = 60 \times \dfrac{1}{150} = ⅖ = 5\overline{)2.0}$ with $\dfrac{0.4}{2\ 0}$

    $x = 0.4$ mg

PROOF: 1 × 0.4 = 0.4

            60 × ¹⁄₁₅₀ = ⅖ = 0.4

☐ **4C** (p. 67)

Use conversion tables for proof.

1.	0.001 g	8.	15 to 16 gtt	15.	5 ml
2.	5000 mg	9.	8 ml	16.	1 ℳ
3.	gr 15	10.	1 ml	17.	Milligrams are smaller than
4.	0.5 g	11.	1000 g		grains (gr i = 60 mg)
5.	gr ¼	12.	0.3 mg	18.	g
6.	1000 ml	13.	180 mg	19.	30 ml
7.	1 oz	14.	30 ml	20.	15 ml

☐ **4D** (p. 67)

REMEMBER: *Know* and *have* go on the *left*.

1. ℥ i:30 ml::℥ 1½:x ml

$$1x = 30 \times 1\frac{1}{2} = \frac{30}{1} \times \frac{3}{2} = 45$$

$x = 45$ ml

PROOF: $30 \times 1\frac{1}{2} = 45$
$1 \times 45 = 45$

2. This is a two-step problem. Must change gr ¹⁄₃₀₀ to mg because that is what you have on hand.

Know   **Want to know**

60 mg:gr i::x mg:gr ¹⁄₃₀₀

$$1x = \frac{1}{300} \times \frac{60}{1} = \frac{1}{5}$$

PROOF: $1 \times \frac{1}{5} = \frac{1}{5}$
$60 \times \frac{1}{300} = \frac{1}{5}$

$x = \frac{1}{5}$ mg   Change ⅕ to a decimal because mg is a metric measure and metric is a decimal system; so: $1 \div 5 = 0.2$ mg.

Have   **Want to know**

0.5 mg:0.5 ml::0.2 mg:x ml
$0.50x = 0.10$
$x = 0.2$ ml   Give 0.2 ml of atropine.

PROOF: $0.50 \times 0.2 = 0.1$
$0.5 \times 0.2 = 0.1$

3. **Know   Want to know**

5 ml:1 ℥::x ml:2 ℥
$x = 10$ ml

PROOF: $5 \times 2 = 10$
$1 \times 10 = 10$

4. **Know**   **Want to know**

60 mg:gr i::x mg:gr ¾   PROOF: $1 \times 45 = 45$
$1x = 60 \times ¾ = 45$ $60 \times ¾ = 45$
$x = 45$ mg

Have   **Want to know**

75 mg:1 ml::45 mg:x ml   PROOF: $1 \times 45 = 45$
$75x = 45$ $75 \times 0.6 = 45$
$x = 0.6$ ml

5. **Know**   **Want to know**

1 g:gr 15::0.6 g:gr x PROOF: $15 \times 0.6 = 9$
$1x = 9$ $1 \times 9 = 9$
$x = $ gr 9

Have   **Want to know**

gr 5:1 tab.::gr 9:x tab.   PROOF: $1 \times 9 = 9$
$5x = 9$ $5 \times 1.8 = 9$
$x = 1.8$ tab.   Give 2 tab. of gr v each tablet.

Can you give ⁸⁄₁₀ of a tablet? Not very easily, so the only thing to do is to give 2 tab. of gr v.

6. **Know**   **Want to know**

60 mg:gr i::650 mg:gr x PROOF: $650 \times 1 = 650$
$60x = 650$ $60 \times 10.8 = 650$
$x = 10$ gr

Have   **Want to know**

gr 5:1 tab.::gr 10.8:x tab.   PROOF: $1 \times 10.8 = 10.8$
$5x = 10.8$ $5 \times 2.1 = 10.8$
$x = 2.1$ tab.   Give 2 tab. of gr 5 each.

7. **Know**   **Want to know**

1 g:gr 15::x g:gr 7½   PROOF: $15 \times 0.5 = 7.5$
$15x = 7½$ $7.5 \times 1 = 7.5$
$x = 0.5$ g

Have   **Want to know**

0.5 g:2.0 cc::0.5 g:x cc   PROOF: $2 \times 0.5 = 1$
$0.5x = 1.0$ $0.5 \times 2 = 1$
$x = 2$ cc (ml)

8. **Have**   **Want to know**

gr 7½:2 ml::gr 5:x ml   PROOF: $2 \times 5 = 10$
$7½x = 2 \times 5 = 10$ $7½ \times 1⅓ = 10$
$x = 1.3$ ml

9. **Know**   **Want to know**

60 mg:1 gr::100 mg:x gr

$60x = 100$

$x = 1.66$ gr

PROOF: $60 \times 1.66 = 99.6$

$1 \times 100 = 100$

Have   **Want to have**

1.5 gr:1 cap::1.6 gr:x capsules

$1.5x = 1.6$

$x = 1.06$ or 1 capsule

(Remember, grains do not convert exactly to metric system: 60–67 mg = 1 gr.)

PROOF: $1.5 \times 1 = 1.5$

$1 \times 1.6 = 1.6$

10. **Know**   **Want to know**

60 mg:1 gr::30 mg:x gr

$60x = 30$

$x = \frac{1}{2}$ gr

PROOF: $60 \times \frac{1}{2} = 30$

$1 \times 30 = 30$

2 gr:1.25 ml::$\frac{1}{2}$ gr:x ml

$2x = 1.25 \times 0.5 = .625$

(Use *either* decimals *or* fractions. Do not mix.)

$x = 0.31$ ml

PROOF: $2 \times 0.31 = 0.62$

$1.25 \times 0.5 = 0.62$

☐ **4E**   (p. 69)

1. **Have**   **Want to know**

gr $\frac{1}{150}$:1 ml::gr $\frac{1}{200}$:x ml

$\frac{1}{150}x = \frac{1}{200} = \frac{1}{200} \div \frac{1}{150} = \frac{1}{200} \times \frac{150}{1} = \frac{3}{4}$ ml

$x = \frac{3}{4}$ ml

Change $\frac{3}{4}$ ml to metric (decimal) $0.75 = 0.8$.

PROOF: $\frac{1}{150} \times \frac{3}{4} = \frac{1}{200}$

$1 \times \frac{1}{200} = \frac{1}{200}$

2. **Have**   **Want to know**

gr $\frac{1}{4}$:1 ml::gr $\frac{1}{6}$:x ml

$\frac{1}{4}x = \frac{1}{6}$

$x = \frac{2}{3}$ ml or $0.66 = 0.7$ ml

Change fraction to metric (decimal).

PROOF: $1 \times \frac{1}{6} = \frac{1}{6}$

$\frac{1}{4} \times \frac{2}{3} = \frac{1}{6}$

3. **Know**   **Want to know**

60 mg:gr i::x mg:gr $\frac{1}{2}$

$1x = 60 \times \frac{1}{2} = 30$

$x = 30$ mg

PROOF: $1 \times 30 = 30$

$60 \times \frac{1}{2} = 30$

Have   **Want to know**

15 mg:1 tab.::30 mg:x tab.

15x = 30

x = 2 tab.

PROOF: 1 × 30 = 30

15 × 2 = 30

4. **Have**   **Want to know**

400,000 U:1 ml::300,000 U:x ml

$$\frac{400,000x}{400,000} = \frac{300,000}{400,000} = \frac{3}{4} = 3 \div 4 = 0.75$$

x = 0.75 ml

PROOF: 1 × 300,000 = 300,000

400,000 × 0.75 = 300,000

Know   **Want to know**

15 ℳ:1 ml::x ℳ:0.75 ml

1x = 15 × 0.75 = 11.25

x = 11 minims

PROOF: 1 × 11 = 11

15 × 0.75 = 11.25

5. **Know**   **Want to know**

1000 mg:1 g::x mg:0.50 g

1x = 500 mg

x = 500 mg

PROOF: 1 × 500 = 500

1000 × 0.50 = 500

Have   **Want to know**

250 mg:1 tab.::500 mg:x tab.

250x = 500

x = 2 tab.

PROOF: 1 × 500 = 500

250 × 2 = 500

6. **Have**   **Want to know**

100 mg:2 ml::75 mg:x ml

100x = 150

x = 1.5 ml

PROOF: 2 × 75 = 150

100 × 1.5 = 150

7. None. We hope you won't give scopolamine when atropine was ordered.

8. **Know**   **Want to know**

1 g:gr 15::x g:gr 7½

15x = 7½

$$1x = \frac{7½}{15} = ½$$

x = 0.5 g

PROOF: 15 × 0.5 = 7.5

1 × 7½ = 7½

Have   **Want to know**

0.25 g:1 tab.::0.5 g:x tab.

$0.25x = 0.5$

$$1x = \frac{0.5}{0.25} = 2$$

$x = 2$ tab.

PROOF: $1 \times 0.5 = 0.5$

$0.25 \times 2 = 0.5$

9. **Know**   **Want to know**

30 ml:1 oz::x ml:½ oz

$x = 30 \times \frac{1}{2} = {}^{30}\!/_2$

$x = 15$ ml

PROOF: $30 \times \frac{1}{2} = 15$

$1 \times 15 = 15$

10. **Know**   **Want to know**

60 mg:1 gr::x mg:$\frac{1}{200}$ gr

$$x = \frac{60}{1} \times \frac{1}{200} = \frac{60\!\!\!/}{200\!\!\!/} = \frac{3}{10}$$

$x = 0.3$ mg

PROOF: $60 \times \frac{1}{200} = 0.3$

$1 \times 0.3 = 0.3$

Have   **Want to know**

0.4 mg:1 ml::0.3 mg:x ml

$$\frac{0.4x}{0.4} = \frac{0.3}{0.4} = 0.75$$

$x = 0.75$ ml

PROOF: $0.4 \times 0.75 = 0.3$

$1 \times 0.3 = 0.3$

CHAPTER 4

Apothecary/Metric System Test (p. 72)

---

1. 0.3 ml
2. 0.66 ml
3. 15 ml
4. 0.37 ml or 0.4
5. 0.5 ml
6. 1 tab
7. 0.67 g
8. 1800 to 2000 mg
9. 450 or 500 mg
10. 45 mg

Medications from powder and crystals

☐ **5A** (p. 76)

1. Add 2.5 ml of sterile water for injection; 330 mg/ml.
   Refrigerated, 96 hrs; room temperature, 24 hrs.

   Have **Want**

   330 mg:1 ml::300 mg:x ml   PROOF: $330 \times 0.9 = 297$

   $330x = 300$ $300 \times 1 = 300$

   $x = 0.9$ ml

   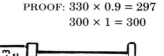

2. Add 5.7 ml of sterile water for injection; 1.5 ml/250 mg.
   Refrigerated, 7 days; room temperature, 3 days.

   Have **Want**

   250 mg:1.5 ml::450 mg:x ml   PROOF: $250 \times 2.7 = 675$

   $250x = 1.5 \times 450 = 675$ $1.5 \times 450 = 675$

   $250x = 675$

   $x = 2.7$ ml

   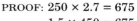

   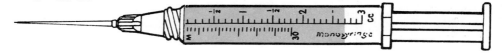

3. Add 3.5 ml diluent.
   The reconstituted medication will yield 250 mg/ml.
   Use within 1 hour—very unstable medication.

   Have **Want**

   250 mg:1 ml::500 mg:x ml   PROOF: $1 \times 500 = 500$

   $250x = 500$ $250 \times 2 = 500$

   $x = 2$ ml

   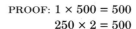
   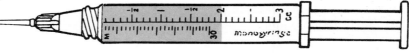

4. Add 5.7 ml sterile water for injection.
   The reconstituted medication will yield 250 mg/1.5 ml.
   Refrigerated, 7 days; room temperature, 3 days.

   Have   **Want**

   250 mg:1.5 ml::300 mg:x ml   PROOF: $1.5 \times 300 = 450$
   $250x = 1.5 \times 300 = 450$ $250 \times 1.8 = 450$
   $x = 1.8$ ml

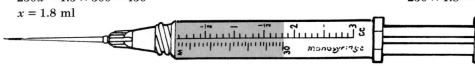

5. Add 5.7 ml of sterile water for injection.
   The reconstituted medication will yield 1 g/2 ml Staphcillin.
   Refrigerated, 4 days; room temperature, 24 hours.

   Have   **Want**

   1000 mg:2 ml::1000 mg:x ml   PROOF: $2 \times 1000 = 2000$
   $1000x = 2 \times 1000 = 2000$ $1000 \times 2 = 2000$
   $x = 2$ ml

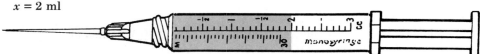

6. 500,000 U/ml
   Add 1.6 ml diluent for injection.
   Refrigerated, 7 days.

   Have   **Want**

   500,000 U:1 ml::750,000 u:x ml   PROOF: $50 \times 1.5 = 75$
   $50x = 1 \times 75 = 75$ $1 \times 75 = 75$
   $50x = 75$
   $x = 1.5$ ml

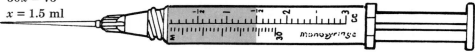

7. Add 2 ml of sterile water for injection.
   The reconstituted medication will yield 1 g/2.6 ml.
   Use medication promptly.

   Have   **Want**

   1000 mg:2.6 ml::750 mg:x ml   PROOF: $1000 \times 1.95 = 1950$
   $1000x = 2.6 \times 750 = 1950$ $2.6 \times 750 = 1950$
   $1000x = 1950$
   $x = 1.95 = 2$ ml

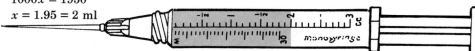

1. **Know**   **Want**

   1 g:1000 mg::x g:500 mg   PROOF: $1000 \times 0.5 = 500$
   $1000x = 500$ $1 \times 500 = 500$
   $x = 0.5$ g

   Have   **Want**

   0.25 g:1.5 ml::0.5 g:x ml   PROOF: $1.5 \times 0.5 = 0.75$
   $0.25x = 1.5 \times 0.5 = 0.75$ $0.25 \times 3 = 0.75$
   $x = 3$ ml

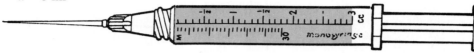

2. Make the 500,000 U per ml solution.

   Have   **Want**

   5̶0̶0̶,̶0̶0̶0̶ U:1 ml::3̶0̶0̶,̶0̶0̶0̶ U:x ml   PROOF: $1 \times 3 = 3$
   $5x = 3$ $5 \times 0.6 = 3$
   $x = 0.6$ ml

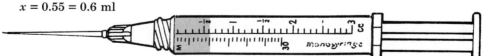

3. **Have**   **Want**

   500 ml:2.2 ml::200 mg:x ml   PROOF: $500 \times 0.88 = 440$
   $500x = 2.2 \times 200 = 440$ $2.2 \times 200 = 440$
   $x = 0.88 = 0.9$ ml

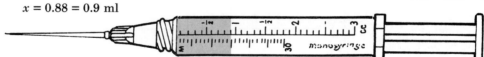

4. **Have**   **Want**

   1 ml:225 mg::x ml:125 mg   PROOF: $1 \times 125 = 125$
   $225x = 125$ $225 \times 0.55 = 123.75$
   $x = 0.55 = 0.6$ ml

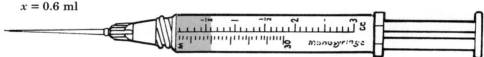

5. Now that you know how to move the decimal three places to the right to change g to mg, this can be a one-step problem.

   Have   **Want**

   1 ml:250 mg::x ml:500 mg   PROOF: $1 \times 500 = 500$
   $250x = 500$ $250 \times 2 = 500$
   $x = 2$ ml

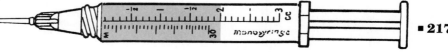

6. You know that 0.50 g = 500 mg. Therefore prepare 2.5 ml of achromycin.

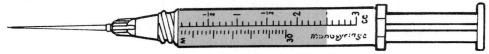

7. You know that 1 g = 1000 mg. Therefore this can be a one-step problem.

Have　　　　**Want**

1000 mg:3 ml::300 mg:x ml　　　　　　　　PROOF: $3 \times 300 = 900$

$1000x = 900$　　　　　　　　　　　　　　　　$1000 \times 0.9 = 900$

$x = 0.9$ ml

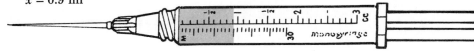

8. **Know**　　　　**Want**

5̶0̶0̶,̶0̶0̶0̶ U:1 ml::1,2̶0̶0̶,̶0̶0̶0̶ U:x ml　　　　PROOF: $1 \times 12 = 12$

$5x = 12$　　　　　　　　　　　　　　　　　　$2.4 \times 5 = 12$

$x = 2.4$ ml will contain 1.2 million U of penicillin

How many ml will be left in the vial?

Vial contains　10.0 ml

Gave　　　　　 2.4 ml

　　　　　　　 7.6 ml remaining in vial

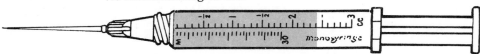

How many units of penicillin will be left in the vial?

Know　　　　**Want**

500,000 U:1 ml::x U:10 ml　　　　　　　PROOF: $1 \times 5{,}000{,}000 = 5{,}000{,}000$

$1x = 10 \times 500{,}000 = 5{,}000{,}000$　　　　　$10 \times 500{,}000 = 5{,}000{,}000$

$x = 5$ million units in entire vial

　5,000,000 units in entire vial

−1,200,000 units given in 2.4 ml

　3,800,000 units left in vial

9. **Have**　　　　**Want**

5̶0̶0̶,̶0̶0̶0̶ U:1 ml::5,0̶0̶0̶,̶0̶0̶0̶ U:x ml　　　PROOF: $5 \times 10 = 50$

$5x = 50$　　　　　　　　　　　　　　　　　　$1 \times 50 = 50$

$x = 10$ ml diluent needed to make 500,000 U/ml

10. **Have**   **Want**

$5\cancel{0}\cancel{0},\cancel{0}\cancel{0}\cancel{0}$ U:1 ml::$8\cancel{0}\cancel{0},\cancel{0}\cancel{0}\cancel{0}$ U:x ml   PROOF: $1 \times 8 = 8$

$5x = 8$ $5 \times 1.6 = 8$

$x = 1.6$ ml

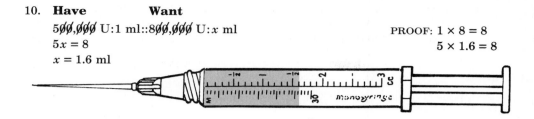

Medications from Powder and Crystals Test   (p. 83)

1. 0.5 ml
   You may cross out zeros in equal amounts on both sides
   of the equation.

2. After diluting with 4 ml of sterile water, give 2.2 ml.

3. 2 ml
   Add 2 ml of distilled water to a vial to make 50,000 U/ml.
   Label vial: date, time, and units per ml.

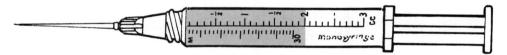

4. Add 2 ml distilled water to vial.   PROOF: $25 \times 4 = 100$
   Each ml of carbenicillin will contain 250,000 U. $1 \times 100 = 100$
   Label vial: date, time, and units/ml.

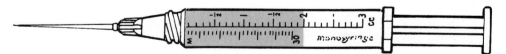

5. $0.6\tfrac{2}{3} = 0.7$ ml   PROOF: $1 \times 4 = 4$

                                     $0.6\tfrac{2}{3} \times 6 = 4$

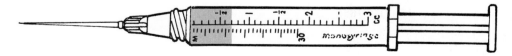

Basic intravenous calculations

□ **6A**   (p. 89)

KNOW: $1 \dfrac{\text{TV}^*}{\text{TT}} = \text{ml/hr}$

$2 \dfrac{\text{D}^*}{\text{M}} \times \text{V} = \text{gtt/min}$

1. *Step 1:* $\dfrac{\text{TV}}{\text{TT}} = \dfrac{1000}{8} = 125 \text{ ml/hr}$

    Step 2: $\dfrac{10}{60} \times \dfrac{125 \text{ ml}}{1} = \dfrac{1}{6} \times \dfrac{125}{1} = \dfrac{125}{6} = 20.8 = 21 \text{ gtt/min}$

2. *Step 2:* $\dfrac{12}{60} \times \dfrac{200}{1} = \dfrac{1}{5} \times \dfrac{200}{1} = \dfrac{200}{5} = 40 \text{ gtt/min}$

3. *Step 2:* $\dfrac{10}{30} \times \dfrac{100}{1} = \dfrac{1}{3} \times \dfrac{100}{1} = \dfrac{100}{3} = 33.3 \text{ or } 33 \text{ gtt/min}$

4. *Step 1:* $\dfrac{1500}{12} = 125 \text{ ml/hr}$

    Step 2: $\dfrac{15}{60} \times \dfrac{125}{1} = \dfrac{1}{4} \times \dfrac{125}{1} = 31.2 \text{ or } 31 \text{ gtt/min}$

5. *Step 2:* $\dfrac{60}{60} \times \dfrac{50}{1} = \dfrac{1}{1} \times \dfrac{50}{1} = \dfrac{50}{1} = 50 \text{ gtt/min}$

6. *Step 1:* $\dfrac{1500}{8} = 188 \text{ ml/hr}$

    Step 2: a. $\dfrac{10}{60} \times \dfrac{188}{1} = \dfrac{1}{6} \times \dfrac{188}{1} = \dfrac{188}{6} = 31.2 \text{ or } 31 \text{ gtt/min}$

    b. $\dfrac{15}{60} = \dfrac{1}{4} \times \dfrac{188}{1} = 47 \text{ gtt/min}$

Always reduce fraction *before* multiplying.

7. *Step 2:* $\dfrac{10}{45} \times \dfrac{75}{1} = \dfrac{750}{45} = 16.6$ or 17 gtt/min

8. *Step 2:* $\dfrac{\overset{2}{\cancel{60}}}{\underset{3}{\cancel{90}}} \times 250 = \dfrac{2}{3} \times \dfrac{250}{1} = \dfrac{500}{3} = 166$ gtt/min

9. *Step 2:* $\dfrac{\overset{3}{\cancel{15}}}{\underset{8}{\cancel{40}}} \times 150 = \dfrac{3}{8} \times \dfrac{150}{1} = \dfrac{450}{8} = 56$ gtt/min

10. *Step 2:* $\dfrac{\overset{1}{\cancel{20}}}{\underset{3}{\cancel{60}}} \times 150 = \dfrac{1}{3} \times \dfrac{150}{1} = \dfrac{150}{3} = 50$ gtt/min

□ **6B** (p. 91)

REMEMBER: $\dfrac{\text{Total volume}}{\text{Total time}} = \text{ml/hr}$

$\dfrac{\text{Drop factor}}{\text{Time (min)}} \times \text{V/hr} = \text{gtt/min}$

1. *Step 1:* $\dfrac{\text{TV}}{\text{TT}} = \dfrac{2000}{24} = 83.3$ ml/hr = 83 ml/hr

2. *Step 1:* $\dfrac{\text{TV}}{\text{TT}} = \dfrac{1500}{8} = 187.5 = 188$ ml/hr

   Step 2: $\dfrac{15}{60} \times \dfrac{188}{1} = \dfrac{\overset{1}{\cancel{15}}}{\underset{4}{\cancel{60}}} \times \dfrac{188}{1} = 47$ gtt/min

3. *Step 1:* $\dfrac{\text{TV}}{\text{TT}} = \dfrac{3000}{24} = 125$ ml/hr

   Step 2: $\dfrac{60}{60} \times \dfrac{125}{1} = 1 \times 125 = 125$ gtt/min

4. *Step 1:* $\dfrac{\text{TV}}{\text{TT}} = \dfrac{500}{4} = 125$ ml/hr

   Step 2: $\dfrac{\overset{1}{\cancel{15}}}{\underset{4}{\cancel{60}}} \times \dfrac{125}{1} = \dfrac{125}{4} = 31.2 = 31$ gtt/min

5. *Step 1:* $\dfrac{\text{TV}}{\text{TT}} = \dfrac{1000}{12} = 83.3 = 83$ ml/hr

   Step 2: $\dfrac{\overset{1}{\cancel{60}}}{\underset{1}{\cancel{60}}} \times \dfrac{83}{1} = \dfrac{83}{1} = 83$ gtt/min

6. Start with step 2 because we already know how many ml per 30 minutes.

   $\dfrac{12}{\underset{3}{\cancel{30}}} \times \dfrac{\overset{10}{\cancel{100}}}{1} = \dfrac{120}{3} = 40$ gtt/min

7. *Step 1:* $\dfrac{\text{TV}}{\text{TT}} = \dfrac{2000}{24} = 83.3 = 83$ ml/hr

   Step 2: $\dfrac{15}{60} \times \dfrac{83}{1} = \dfrac{\overset{1}{\cancel{15}}}{\underset{4}{\cancel{60}}} \times \dfrac{83}{1} = \dfrac{83}{4} = 20.75 = 21$ gtt/min

8. *Step 1:* $\dfrac{\text{TV}}{\text{TT}} = \dfrac{250}{10} = 25$ ml/hr

   Step 2: $\dfrac{\overset{1}{\cancel{60}}}{\underset{1}{\cancel{60}}} \times \dfrac{25}{1} = 25$ gtt/min

9. *Step 1:* $\dfrac{\text{TV}}{\text{TT}} = \dfrac{1500}{12} = 125$ ml/hr

   Step 2: $\dfrac{\overset{1}{\cancel{15}}}{\underset{4}{\cancel{60}}} \times \dfrac{125}{1} = \dfrac{125}{4} = 31$ gtt/min

10.   MEMORIZE: $\dfrac{TV}{TT}$ = ml/hr

$$\frac{\text{Drop factor}}{\text{Time (min)}} \times \text{V/hr} = \text{gtt/min} \text{ or } \frac{D}{M} \times V = \text{gtt/min}$$

☐ **6C**   (p. 93)

REMEMBER: *Step 1:* $\dfrac{TV}{TT}$ = ml/hr

$$\text{Step 2: } \frac{D}{M} \times V = \text{gtt/min}$$

1.   *Step 2:* $\dfrac{1\cancel{0}}{6\cancel{0}} \times 100 = \dfrac{100}{6} = 16.6 = 17$ gtt/min

2.   *Step 1:* $\dfrac{TV}{TT} = \dfrac{1000}{6} = 166.6 = 167$ ml/hr

   Step 2: $\dfrac{15}{60} \times \dfrac{167}{1} = \dfrac{\overset{1}{\cancel{15}}}{\underset{4}{\cancel{60}}} \times \dfrac{167}{1} = \dfrac{167}{4} = 41.75 = 42$ gtt/min

3.   *Step 2:* $\dfrac{10}{30} \times \dfrac{50}{1} = \dfrac{1\cancel{0}}{3\cancel{0}} \times \dfrac{50}{1} = \dfrac{50}{3} = 16.6 = 17$ gtt/min

4.   *Step 2:* $\dfrac{60}{60} \times \dfrac{100}{1} = \dfrac{\overset{1}{\cancel{60}}}{\underset{1}{\cancel{60}}} \times \dfrac{100}{1} = 100$ gtt/min

5.   *Step 1:* $\dfrac{TV}{TT} = \dfrac{2000}{12} = 166.6 = 167$ ml/hr

   Step 2: $\dfrac{60}{60} \times \dfrac{167}{1} = \dfrac{\overset{1}{\cancel{60}}}{\underset{1}{\cancel{60}}} \times \dfrac{167}{1} = 167$ gtt/min

6.   *Step 2:* $\dfrac{12}{30} \times \dfrac{100}{1} = \dfrac{12}{3\cancel{0}} \times \dfrac{10\cancel{0}}{1} = \dfrac{120}{3} = 40$ gtt/min

7. *Step 1:* $\dfrac{\text{TV}}{\text{TT}} = \dfrac{1500}{24} = 62.5 = 63 \text{ ml/hr}$

   Step 2: $\dfrac{10}{60} \times \dfrac{63}{1} = \dfrac{1\cancel{0}}{6\cancel{0}} \times \dfrac{63}{1} = \dfrac{63}{6} \times 10.5 = 11 \text{ gtt/min}$

8. *Step 1:* $\dfrac{\text{TV}}{\text{TT}} = \dfrac{500}{8} = 62.5 = 63 \text{ ml/hr}$

   Step 2: $\dfrac{60}{60} \times \dfrac{63}{1} = \dfrac{\cancel{60}^{1}}{\cancel{60}_{1}} \times \dfrac{63}{1} = 63 \text{ gtt/min}$

9. *Step 2:* $\dfrac{15}{60} \times 75 = \dfrac{1}{4} \times \dfrac{75}{1} = \dfrac{75}{4} = 18.7 = 19 \text{ gtt/min}$

10. *Step 2:* $\dfrac{20}{60} \times 85 = \dfrac{1}{3} \times \dfrac{85}{1} = \dfrac{85}{3} = 28.3 = 28 \text{ gtt/min}$

☐ **6D** (p. 96)

1. $\dfrac{15}{60} \times \dfrac{100}{1} = \dfrac{1}{4} \times \dfrac{100}{1} = \dfrac{100}{4} = 25 \text{ gtt/min}$

2. $\dfrac{15}{20} \times \dfrac{50}{1} = \dfrac{\cancel{15}^{3}}{\cancel{20}_{4}} \times \dfrac{50}{1} = \dfrac{150}{4} = 37.5 = 38 \text{ gtt/min}$

3. $\dfrac{60}{30} \times \dfrac{50}{1} = \dfrac{\cancel{60}^{2}}{\cancel{30}_{1}} \times \dfrac{50}{1} = 100 \text{ gtt/min}$

4. $\dfrac{12}{60} \times \dfrac{100}{1} = \dfrac{\cancel{12}^{1}}{\cancel{60}_{5}} \times \dfrac{100}{1} = \dfrac{100}{5} = 20 \text{ gtt/min}$

5.

Know	**Want to know**

   Step 1: 20 gtt:1 ml::x gtt:250 ml

   $\qquad\qquad x = 20 \times 250 = 5000$

   $\qquad\qquad x = 5000 \text{ gtt in 250 ml}$

	Know	**Want to know**

Step 2: 60 gtt:1 minute::5000 gtt:x minutes

$$60x = 5000 = \frac{5000}{60}$$

$x = 83.3$ minutes = 1 hour, 23 minutes

6.

	Know	**Want to know**

Step 1: 15 gtt:1 ml::x gtt:2000 ml

$x = 15 \times 2000 = 30{,}000$

$x = 30{,}000$ gtt in 2000 ml

	Know	**Want to know**

Step 2: 40 gtt:1 minute::30,000 gtt:x minutes

$$40x = 30{,}000 = \frac{30{,}00\cancel{0}}{4\cancel{0}} = 750$$

$x = 750$ minutes = 12½ hours to infuse

7.

$$\frac{\overset{3}{\cancel{60}}}{\underset{2}{\cancel{40}}} \times 150 = \frac{450}{2} = 225 \text{ gtt/min is the fastest rate}$$

$$\frac{\cancel{60}}{\cancel{60}} \times 150 = 150 \text{ gtt/min is the slowest rate}$$

8.

	Know	**Want to know**

Step 1: 15 gtt:1 ml::x gtt:1000 ml

$x = 15 \times 1000 = 15{,}000$

$x = 15{,}000$ gtt in 1000 ml

	Know	**Want to know**

Step 2: 40 gtt:1 minute::15,000 gtt:x minutes

$40x = 15{,}000$

$x = 375$ minutes = 6 hours, 15 minutes to infuse

9.

$$\frac{\overset{2}{\cancel{60}}}{\underset{1}{\cancel{30}}} \times 100 = 200 \text{ gtt/min}$$

10.   **Know**   **Want to know**

Step 1:   60 gtt:1 ml::x gtt:200 ml
            $x = 60 \times 200 = 12{,}000$
            $x = 12{,}000$ gtt in 200 ml

           Know   **Want to know**

Step 2:   50 gtt:1 minute::12,000 gtt:x minutes
            $50x = 12{,}000$
            $x = 240$ minutes $= 4$ hours

☐ **6E**   (p. 98)

1. $\dfrac{\overset{1}{\cancel{20}}}{\underset{3}{\cancel{60}}} \times 40 = \dfrac{40}{3} = 13$ gtt/min

2. $\dfrac{\overset{1}{\cancel{15}}}{\underset{4}{\cancel{60}}} \times 80 = \dfrac{80}{4} = 20$ gtt/min

    Know   **Want to know**

    80 ml:1 hr::x ml:24 hr
    $x = 80 \times 24 = 1920$
    $x = 1920$ ml in 24 hr

3. $\dfrac{60}{60} \times 125 = 125$ gtt/min and 125 ml/hr

4. $\dfrac{3000}{24} = 125$ ml/hr $= 125$ gtt/min

5. $\dfrac{2000}{24} = 83.3 = 83$ ml/hr

    $\dfrac{\overset{1}{\cancel{20}}}{\underset{3}{\cancel{60}}} \times 83 = \dfrac{83}{3} = 27.6 = 28$ gtt/min

CHAPTER 6

Basic Intravenous Calculations Test   (p. 99)

1. 125ml/hr
    31 gtt/min
    (Step 1)
2. 17 gtt/min
    (Step 2)
3. 83 ml/hr
    17 gtt/min
    (Step 1)
4. 150 ml/hr
    150 gtt/min
    (Step 1)

5. 83 ml/hr
    14 gtt/min
    (Step 1)
6. 125 ml/hr
    31 gtt/min
    (Step 1)
7. 125 ml/hr
    125 gtt/min
    (Step 1)

8. 83 ml/hr
    21 gtt/min
    (Step 1)
9. 83 ml/hr
    83 gtt/min
    (Step 1)
10. 167 gtt/min
    (Step 2)

INSULIN

☐ **7A** (p. 108)

1.	27 U	4.	0.44 U
2.	68 U	5.	32 U
3.	16 U	6.	78 U

☐ **7B** (p. 109)

1. Total units: 55
    Onset/duration: 15 min-24 hr
    Peak: 2-12 hr
    Labels: D and I
    Which drawn up first: E
    Source: Beef and pork

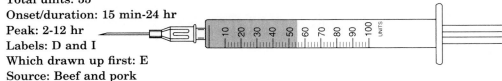

2. Total units: 43
    Onset/duration: 30 min-24 hr
    Peak: 2-12 hr
    Labels: A and H
    Source: Recombinant DNA

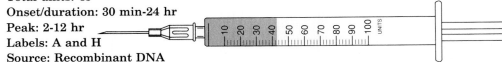

3. Total units: 23
    Onset/duration: 30 min-24 hr
    Peak: 2-12 hr
    Labels: C and L
    Source: Pork and beef

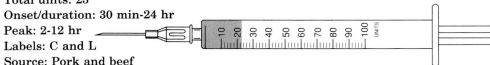

4. Total units: 57
    Onset/duration: 15 min-24 hr
    Peak: 2-12 hr
    Labels: B and L
    Source: Beef/pork and Pork (use a beef/pork source)

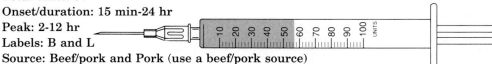

5. Total units: 68
    Onset/duration: 15 min-24 hr
    Peak: 2-12 hr
    Labels: B and K
    Source: Beef/pork and beef/pork

6. Total units: 50
    Onset/duration: 30 min-24 hr
    Peak: 2-12 hr
    Labels: A and H
    Source: Human and human

7. Total units: 46
   Onset/duration: 15 min-24 hr
   Peak: 2-12 hr
   Labels: C and J
   Source: Pork and pork

8. Total units: 64
   Onset/duration: 15 min-24 hr
   Peak: 2-12 hr
   Labels: D and K
   Source: Beef/pork and beef/pork

9. Total units: 42
   Onset/duration: 30 min-24 hr
   Peak: 2-15 hr
   Labels: E and M
   Source: Human and Human

10. Total units: 76
    Onset/duration: 30 min-24 hr
    Peak: 2-12 hr
    Labels: F and M
    Source: Human and human

□ **7C** (p. 112)

1. 35 U

2. 20 U Onset 15-30 min
3. 44 U Peak 6-12 hr

4. 65 U Duration 6-8 hr
5. 20 U Onset 15-30 min

6. 60 U 30 min-24 hr

7. 15 U One RN

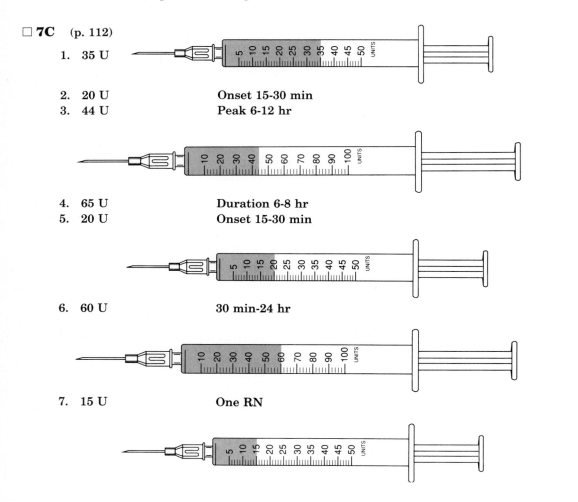

8. Peak 14-24 hr   Duration 28-36 hr

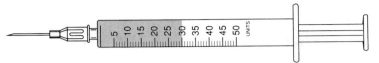

9. Onset 15-30 min   Peak 2-5

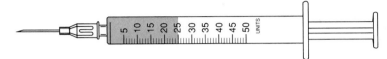

10. Peak 14-24 hr   Duration 28-36 hr

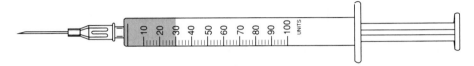

☐ **7D**   (p. 116)

1. **Have   Want to know**

   100 U:150 ml::10 U:x ml   PROOF: $100 \times 15 = 1500$
   $100x = 150 \times 10 = 1500$ $150 \times 10 = 1500$
   $100x = 1500$
   $x = 15$ ml/hr = 10 U insulin
        15 gtt/min = microdrip

   Know   Want to know

   15 ml:1 hour::150 ml:x hr   PROOF: $15 \times 10 = 150$
   $15x = 150$ $1 \times 150 = 150$
   $x = 10$ hr to infuse 100 U insulin

2. **Have   Want to know**

   50 ml:50 U::x ml:8 U   PROOF: $50 \times 8 = 400$
   $50x = 50 \times 8 = 400$ $50 \times 8 = 400$
   $50x = 400$
   $x = 8$ ml/hr = 8 U of insulin
        microdrip = 8 gtt/min

   Know   Want to know

   8 ml:1 hr::50 ml:x hr   PROOF: $8 \times 6.25 = 50$
   $8x = 50$ $1 \times 50 = 50$
   $x = 6.25$ hr to infuse 50 U insulin

3. **Have**   **Want to know**

50 ml:75 U::x ml:5 U   PROOF: $50 \times 5 = 250$

$75x = 50 \times 5 = 250$ $75 \times 3.33 = 249.75$

$75x = 250$

$x = 3.33$ ml/hr = 5 U

    (3 gtt/min for microdrip)

Know   **Want to know**

3 ml:1 hr::50 ml:x hr   PROOF: $3 \times 16.6 = 49.8$

$3x = 50$ $1 \times 50 = 50$

$x = 16.6$ hr to infuse

4. **Have**   **Want to know**

100 ml:120 U::x ml:10 U   PROOF: $120 \times 8.33 = 999.6$

$120x = 100 \times 10 = 1000$ $100 \times 10 = 1000$

$120x = 1000$

$x = 8.33$ ml/hr to deliver 10 U of insulin

    (8 gtt/hr for microdrip)

Know   **Want to know**

8 ml:1 hr::100 ml:x hr   PROOF: $8 \times 12.5 = 100$

$8x = 1 \times 100 = 100$ $1 \times 100 = 100$

$8x = 100$

$x = 12.5$ hr to infuse 120 U of regular insulin

5. **Have**   **Want to know**

150 ml:150 U::x ml:12 U   PROOF: $150 \times 12 = 1800$

$150x = 150 \times 12 = 1800$ $12 \times 150 = 1800$

$150x = 1800$

$x = 12$ ml/hr to deliver 12 U of insulin/hr

    (12 gtt/min microdrip)

Know   **Want to know**

12 ml:1 hr::150 ml:x hr   PROOF: $12 \times 12.5 = 150$

$12x = 150$ $1 \times 150 = 150$

$x = 12.5$ hr to infuse 150 U of regular insulin

6. **Have**   **Want to know**

500 ml:24 hr::x ml:1 hr   PROOF: $24 \times 20.8 = 499.2$

$24x = 500$ $1 \times 500 = 500$

$x = 20.8 = 21$ ml/hr = 24 gtt/min microdrip

Know   **Want to know**

50 U:24 hr::x U:1 hr   PROOF: $24 \times 2 = 48$

$24x = 50$ $50 \times 1 = 50$

$x = 2$ U/hr

7. **Have**   **Want to know**

    100 U:24 hr::x U:1 hr   PROOF: $24 \times 4.1 = 98.4$
    $24x = 100$ $100 \times 1 = 100$
    $x = 4.1$ U/hr

    Know   **Want to know**

    250 ml:24 hr::x ml:1 hr   PROOF: $24 \times 10.4 = 249.6$
    $24x = 250$ $250 \times 1 = 250$
    $x = 10.4 = 10$ ml/hr = 10 gtt/min microdrip

8. **Have**   **Want to know**

    50 ml:24 hr::x ml:1 hr   PROOF: $50 \times 1 = 50$
    $24x = 50$ $24 \times 2.08 = 49.92$
    $x = 2$ ml/hr = 2 gtt/min microdrip

    Know   **Want to know**

    100 U:24 hr::x U:1 hr   PROOF: $24 \times 4.16 = 99.84$
    $24x = 100$ $100 \times 1 = 100$
    $x = 4.16$ U/hr

9. **Have**   **Want to know**

    100 ml:12 hr::x ml:1 hr   PROOF: $12 \times 8.33 = 99.6$
    $12x = 100$ $100 \times 1 = 100$
    $x = 8.33 = 8$ ml/hr = 8 gtt/min microdrip

    Know   **Want to know**

    25 U:100 ml::x U:8 ml   PROOF: $100 \times 2 = 200$
    $100x = 25 \times 8 = 200$ $25 \times 8 = 200$
    $x = 2$ U/ml or 2 U/hr

10. **Have**   **Want to know**

    65 U:24 hr::x U:1 hr   PROOF: $24 \times 2.7 = 64.8$
    $24x = 65 \times 1 = 65$ $65 \times 1 = 65$
    $24x = 65$
    $x = 2.7$ U/hr

    Know   **Want to know**

    150 ml:24 hr::x ml:1 hr   PROOF: $24 \times 6.25 = 150$
    $24x = 150$ $150 \times 1 = 150$
    $x = 6.25$ ml/hr = 6 gtt/min microdrip

Insulin Test   (p. 119)

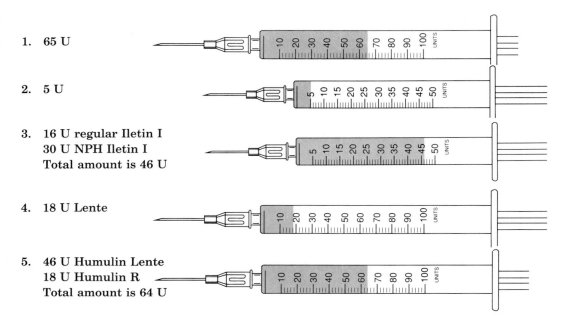

1. 65 U

2. 5 U

3. 16 U regular Iletin I
   30 U NPH Iletin I
   Total amount is 46 U

4. 18 U Lente

5. 46 U Humulin Lente
   18 U Humulin R
   Total amount is 64 U

6. **Know**   **Want to know**
   500 ml:250 U::x ml:10 U
   $250x = 500 \times 10 = 5000$
   $25\emptyset x = 500\emptyset$
   $x = 20$ ml/hr = 10 U = 20 gtt/min microdrip

   PROOF: $500 \times 10 = 5000$
   $250 \times 20 = 5000$

   Know   **Want to know**
   20 ml:1 hour::500 ml:x hours
   $20x = 500$
   $x = 25$ hours to infuse

   PROOF: $1 \times 500 = 500$
   $20 \times 25 = 500$

7. **Know**   **Want to know**
   250 ml:100 U::x ml:6 U
   $100x = 250 \times 6 = 1500$
   $x = 15$ ml/hr = 15 gtt/min to deliver 6 U insulin

   PROOF: $250 \times 6 = 1500$
   $6 \times 250 = 1500$

   Know   **Want to know**
   15 ml:1 hour::250 ml:x hours
   $15x = 250$
   $x = 16.6$ hours

   PROOF: $1 \times 250 = 250$
   $15 \times 16.6 = 249$

8. **Know**   **Want to know**

100 U:250 ml::8 U:x ml   PROOF: $250 \times 8 = 2000$

$100x = 250 \times 8 = 2000$ $100 \times 20 = 2000$

$1\cancel{00}x = 20\cancel{00}$

$x = 20$ ml/hr $= 8$ U insulin $= 20$ gtt/min

Know   **Want to know**

20 ml:1 hour::250 ml:x hours   PROOF: $20 \times 12.5 = 250$

$20x = 250$ $1 \times 250 = 250$

$x = 12.5$ hours to infuse

9. **Know**   **Want to know**

200 ml:100 U::x ml:7 U   PROOF: $200 \times 7 = 1400$

$100x = 200 \times 7 = 1400$ $100 \times 14 = 1400$

$1\cancel{00}x = 14\cancel{00}$

$x = 14$ ml/hr $= 14$ gtt/min $= 7$ units of insulin

Know   **Want to know**

14 ml:1 hour::200 ml:x hours   PROOF: $14 \times 14.2 = 198.8$

$14x = 200$ $1 \times 200 = 200$

$x = 14.2$ hours to infuse

10. **Know**   **Want to know**

500 ml:100 U::x ml:9 U   PROOF: $500 \times 9 = 4500$

$100x = 500 \times 9 = 4500$ $100 \times 45 = 4500$

$1\cancel{00}x = 45\cancel{00}$

$x = 45$ ml/hr $= 45$ gtt/min to deliver 9 U insulin

Know   **Want to know**

45 ml:1 hour::500 ml:x hours   PROOF: $45 \times 11.1 = 499.5$

$45x = 500$ $1 \times 500 = 500$

$x = 11.1$ hours to infuse

CHAPTER 8

Heparin

☐ **8A**   (p. 122)

1. **Have**   **Want**

10,~~000~~ U:1 ml::7,~~000~~ U:x ml   PROOF: $1 \times 7000 = 7000$

$10x = 7$ $10,000 \times 0.7 = 7000$

$x = 0.7$ ml

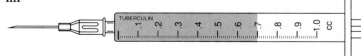

2. **Have**   **Want**

20,~~000~~ U:1 ml::15,~~000~~ U:x ml   PROOF: $1 \times 15,000 = 15,000$

$20x = 15$ $20,000 \times 0.75 = 15,000$

$x = 0.75$ ml

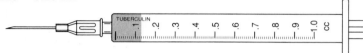

3. **Have**   **Want**

20,~~000~~ U:1 ml::25~~00~~ U:x ml   PROOF: $200 \times 0.125 = 25$

$200x = 25$ $1 \times 25 = 25$

$x = 0.125 = 0.13$ ml

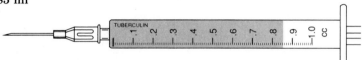

4. **Have**   **Want**

20,~~000~~ U:1 ml::17,~~000~~ U:x ml $\left.\begin{array}{l} \\ \\ \\ \end{array}\right\}$ use the 20,000 U/ml strength   PROOF: $1 \times 17 = 17$

$20x = 17$ $20 \times 0.85 = 17$

$x = 0.85$ ml

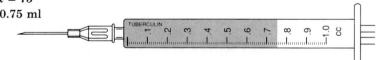

5. **Have**   **Want**

10,~~000~~ U:1 ml::75~~00~~ U:x ml   PROOF: $1 \times 75 = 75$

$100x = 1 \times 75 = 75$ $100 \times 0.75 = 75$

$100x = 75$

$x = 0.75$ ml

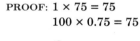

□ **8B**   (p. 124)

1. **Know**   **Want to know**

20,~~000~~ U:1000 ml::1~~000~~ U:x ml   PROOF: $20,000 \times 50 = 1,000,000$

$20x = 1000 \times 1 = 1000$ $1000 \times 1000 = 1,000,000$

$2\cancel{0}x = 100\cancel{0}$

$x = 50$ ml/hr $= 1000$ U heparin

$\dfrac{60}{60} \times 50 = 50$ gtt/min microdrip

2. $\dfrac{1000}{12} = 83.3 = 83$ ml/hr

   $\dfrac{60}{60} \times 83 = 83$ gtt/min microdrip

   Know   **Want to know**

   20,000 U:12 hours::x U:1 hour   PROOF: 20,000 × 1 = 20,000

   $12x = 20,000$ 12 × 1666 = 19,992

   $x = 1666$ U/hr

3. **Know**   **Want to know**

   200Ø̶Ø̶ U:1000 ml::15Ø̶Ø̶ U:x ml   PROOF: 200 × 75 = 15,000

   2Ø̶Ø̶$x = 150$Ø̶Ø̶   1000 × 15 = 15,000

   $x = 75$ ml/hr = 1500 U heparin

   $\dfrac{60}{60} \times 75 = 75$ gtt/min microdrip

4. **Know**   **Want to know**

   10,000 U:15 hrs::x U:1 hr   PROOF: 15 × 666 = 9990

   $15x = 1 \times 10,000 = 10,000$ 10,000 × 1 = 10,000

   $x = 666$ U/hr

5. **Know**   **Want to know**

   10,000 U:500 ml::1200 U:x ml   PROOF: 500 × 12 = 6000

   $100x = 500 \times 12 = 6000$ 100 × 60 = 6000

   $100x = 6000$

   $x = 60$ ml/hr = 1200 U heparin

          60 gtt/min microdrip

6. **Have**   **Want to know**

   50,Ø̶Ø̶Ø̶ U:1000 ml::2,Ø̶Ø̶Ø̶ U:x ml   PROOF: 50 × 40 = 2000

   $50x = 1000 \times 2 = 2000$ 1000 × 2 = 2000

   5Ø̶$x = 200$Ø̶

   $x = 40$ ml/hr = 40 gtt/min

7. **Have**   **Want to know**

   25,Ø̶Ø̶Ø̶ U:500 ml::1Ø̶Ø̶Ø̶ U:x ml   PROOF: 25 × 20 = 500

   $25x = 500$ 500 × 1 = 500

   $x = 20$ ml/hr = 20 gtt/min

8. **Have**   **Want to know**

   25,0Ø̶Ø̶ U:500 ml::13Ø̶Ø̶ U:x ml   PROOF: 25 × 260 = 6500

   $250x = 500 \times 13 = 6500$ 500 × 13 = 6500

   $250x = 6500$

   $x = 26$ ml/hr = 26 gtt/min

9. **Have** **Want to know**

25,0~~00~~ U:250 ml::1,8~~00~~ U:x ml   PROOF: 250 × 18 = 4500

$250x = 250 \times 18 = 4500$ 250 × 18 = 4500

$25\cancel{0}x = 450\cancel{0}$

$x = 18$ ml/hr = 18 gtt/min

10. **Have** **Want to know**

20,~~000~~ U:250 ml::1~~000~~ U:x ml   PROOF: 20 × 12.5 = 250

$2\cancel{0}x = 25\cancel{0}$ 250 × 1 = 250

$x = 12.5$ ml/hr = 13 gtt/min

Heparin Test   (p. 127)

---

1. 0.8 ml
2. 0.25 ml
3. 0.2 ml using the 10,000 U/ml strength
4. 0.35 ml using the 20,000 U/ml strength
5. 0.6 ml

6. **Have** **Want to know**

20,0~~00~~ U:500 ml::7~~00~~ U:x ml   PROOF: 200 × 17.5 = 3500

$200x = 500 \times 7 = 3500$ 500 × 7 = 3500

$2\cancel{00}x = 35\cancel{00}$

$x = 17.5$ ml/hr = 18 gtt/min

7. **Have** **Want to know**

25,0~~00~~ U:500 ml::15~~00~~ U:x ml   PROOF: 250 × 30 = 7500

$25\cancel{0}x = 500 \times 15 = 750\cancel{0}$ 500 × 15 = 7500

$25x = 750$

$x = 30$ ml/hr = 30 gtt/min

8. **Have** **Want to know**

1000 ml:24 hr::x ml:1 hr   PROOF: 24 × 41.6 = 998.4

$24x = 1000$ 1000 × 1 = 1000

$x = 41.6$ ml/hr = 42 gtt/min

  Know **Want to know**

25000 U:24 hr::x U:1 hr   PROOF: 1 × 25000 = 25000

$24x = 25000$ 24 × 1041.6 = 24998.4

$x = 1041.6$ U/hr

9. **Have**   **Want to know**

500 ml:25,0̸0̸0̸ U::x ml:18̸0̸0̸ U   PROOF: $250 \times 36 = 9000$

$250x = 500 \times 18 = 9000$ $500 \times 18 = 9000$

$25̸0̸x = 900̸0̸$

$x = 36$ ml/hr $= 36$ gtt/min

10. Give 0.1 ml of purified protein derivative (PPD) intradermally. A TB syringe is always used for accuracy.

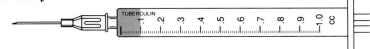

CHAPTER 9

Children's dosages

☐ **9A**   (p. 135)

1. a. 14 lb = approximately 7 kg
   This is a one-step problem.
   Step 1: lb to kg

   Know   **Want to know**

   2.2 lb:1 kg::14 lb:x kg   PROOF: $2.2 \times 6.363^* = 13.99$ or 14

   $2.2x = 14 \times 1$ $1 \times 14 = 14$

   $x = 14/2.2 = 6.363$ or 6.4 kg

   b. 12 lb, 2 oz = approximately 6 kg.
   This is a two-step problem
   Step 1: oz to lb

   Know   **Want to know**

   16 oz:1 lb::2 oz:x lb   PROOF: $16 \times 0.125 = 2$

   $16x = 2 \times 1$ $1 \times 2 = 2$

   $x = 2/16$ or 0.125
   Total weight: 12.125 or 12.1 lb

   Step 2: lb to kg

   Know   **Want to know**

   2.2 lb:1 kg::12.1 lb:x kg   PROOF: $2.2 \times 5.5 = 12.1$

   2.2 lb = 12.1 $1 \times 12.1 = 12.1$

   $x = 12.1/2.2 = 5.5$ kg

---

*Proofs are inexact due to rounding. For exact proofs, need to carry fractions to three decimal places in most cases.

c. 10 lb = approximately 5 kg
This is a one-step problem
Step 1: lb to kg

Know   **Want to know**

2.2 lb:1 kg::10 lb:x kg   PROOF: 2.2 × 4.5 = 9.9 or 10
2.2x = 10 × 1   1 × 10 = 10
x = 10/2.2 = 4.54 or 4.5 kg

d. 7 lb, 6 oz = approximately 3.5 kg
This is a two-step problem
Step 1: oz to lb

Know   **Want to know**

16 oz:1 lb::6 oz:x lb   PROOF: 16 × 0.37 = 5.92 or 6*
16x = 6 × 1   1 × 6 = 6
x = 6/16 = 0.37 lb
Total weight = 7.4 lb

Step 2: lb to kg

Know   **Want to know**

2.2 lb:1 kg::7.4 lb:x kg   PROOF: 2.2 × 3.36 = 7.39 or 7.4
2.2x = 7.4 × 1   1 × 7.4 = 7.4
x = 7.4/2.2 = 3.36 or 3.4 kg

e. 15 lb, 8 oz = approximately 7.5 kg
This is a two-step problem
Step 1: oz to lb

Know   **Want to know**

16 oz:1 lb::8 oz:x lb   PROOF: 16 × 0.5 = 8
16x = 8 × 1   1 × 8 = 8
x = 8/16 = 0.5 lb

Step 2: lb to kg

Know   **Want to know**

2.2 lb:1 kg::15.5 lb:x kg   PROOF: 2.2 × 7 = 15.48 or 15.5
2.2x = 15.5 × 1   1 × 15.5 = 15.5
x = 15.5/2.2 = 7.04 or 7.0 kg

---

*Proofs are inexact due to rounding. For exact proofs, need to round to three decimal places in most cases.

2. a. 150 mg × 3 = 450 mg
    b. 200 mg × 4 = 800 mg
    c. 400 μg × 6 = 2400 μg or 2.4 mg
    d. 50 mg × 3 = 150 mg
    e. 750 μg × 2 = 1500 μg or 1.5 mg

3. a. **Know**   **Want to know**

     10 mg:1 kg::x mg:5 kg   PROOF: 10 × 5 = 50

     x = 5 × 10 or 50 mg   1 × 5 = 50

    b. This is a two-step problem.

     Step 1: Low dose

     Know   **Want to know**

     5 mg:1 kg::x mg:7.3 kg   PROOF: 5 × 7.3 = 36.5

     x = 7.3 × 5   1 × 36.5 = 36.5

     x = 36.5 mg

     Step 2: High dose

     Know   **Want to know**

     8 mg:1 kg::x:7.3 kg   PROOF: 8 × 7.3 = 58.4

     x = 7.5 × 8   1 × 58.4 = 58.4

     x = 58.4 mg

     Answer: Safe-dose range is 36.5 to 58.4 mg.

    c. This is a three-step problem

     Step 1: lb to kg

     8 lb = approximately 4 kg

     Know   **Want to know**

     2.2 lb:1 kg::8 lb:x kg   PROOF: 2.2 × 3.6 = 7.92 or 8

     2.2x = 8 × 1   1 × 8 = 8

     x = 8/2.2 or 3.63 or 3.6 kg

     Step 2: Low dose

     Know   **Want to know**

     6 mg:1 kg::x mg:3.6 kg   PROOF: 6 × 3.6 = 21.6

     x = 3.6 × 6   1 × 21.6 = 21.6

     x = 21.6 mg

     Step 3: High dose

     Know   **Want to know**

     8 mg:1 kg::x mg:3.6 kg   PROOF: 8 × 3.6 = 28.8

     x = 3.6 × 8   1 × 28.8 = 28.8

     x = 28.8 mg

     Answer: Safe-dose range is 21.6 to 28.8 mg.

d. This is a four-step problem
   5 lb, 8 oz = approximately 2.5 kg
   Step 1: oz to lb

   Know   Want to know
   16 oz:1 lb::8 oz:x lb   PROOF: 16 × 0.5 = 8
   $16x = 8 × 1$ 1 × 8 = 8
   $x = 8/16 = 0.5$ lb

   Step 2: lb to kg

   Know   Want to know
   2.2 lb:1 kg::5.5 lb:x kg   PROOF: 2.2 × 2.5 = 5.5
   $2.2x = 5.5 × 1$ 1 × 5.5 = 5.5
   $x = 5.5/2.2 = 2.5$ kg

   Step 3: Low dose

   Know   Want to know
   3 mg:1 kg::x mg:2.5 kg   PROOF: 3 × 2.5 = 7.5
   $1x = 2.5 × 3$ 1 × 7.5 = 7.5
   $x = 7.5$ mg

   Step 4: High dose

   Know   Want to know
   6 mg:1 kg::x mg:2.5 kg   PROOF: 6 × 2.5 = 15
   $1x = 2.5 × 6$ 1 × 15 = 15
   $x = 15$ mg

   Answer: Safe-dose range is 7.5 to 15 mg.

e. This is a four-step problem
   4 lb, 6 oz = approximately 2 kg
   Step 1: oz to lb

   Know   Want to know
   16 oz:1 lb::6 oz:x lb   PROOF: 16 × 0.37 = 5.92 or 6
   $16x = 6 × 1$ 1 × 6 = 6
   $x = 6/16 = 0.37$ or 0.4 lb

   Step 2: lb to kg

   Know   Want to know
   2.2 lb:1 kg::4.4 lb:x kg   PROOF: 2.2 × 2 = 4.4
   $2.2x = 4.4 × 1$ 1 × 4.4 = 4.4
   $x = 4.4/2.2 = 2$ kg

Step 3: Low dose

Know   **Want to know**

200 μg:1 kg::x μg:2 kg   PROOF: 200 × 2 = 400
1x = 2 × 200   1 × 400 = 400
x = 400 μg or 0.4 mg

Step 4: High dose

Know   **Want to know**

400 μg:1 kg::x μg:2 kg   PROOF: 400 × 2 = 800
1x = 2 × 400   1 × 800 = 800
x = 800 μg or 0.8 mg

Answer: Safe-dose range is 400 to 800 μg or 0.4 to 0.8 mg

4.   a.   0.15 m²   5.   a.   0.28/1.7 × 125 mg = 20.5 or 21 mg
     b.   0.20 m²   b.   0.32/1.7 × 250 mg = 47.5 or 48 mg
     c.   0.27 m²   c.   0.45/1.7 × 5 mg = 1.3 or 1 mg
     d.   0.60 m²   d.   0.80/1.7 × 500 mg = 235 mg
     e.   1.10 m²   e.   1.27/1.7 × 100 mg = 74.7 or 75 mg

□ **9B**   (p. 137)

1.   Estimated wt: 12
     Weight in kg:

Know   **Want to know**

2.2 lb:1 kg::25.4 lb:x kg   PROOF: 2.2 × 11.54 = 25.38 or 25.4
2.2x = 25.4   1 × 25.4 = 25.4
x = 11.54 or 11.5 kg

Recommended dose—24 hours:

Know   **Want to know**

10:1:: x mg:11.5 kg   PROOF: 10 × 11.5 = 115
x = 10 × 11.5 or 115 mg—low safe dose   1 × 115 = 115

Know   **Want to know**

30:1:: x:11.5   PROOF: 30 × 11.5 = 345
1x = 30 × 11.5   1 × 345 = 345
x = 345 mg—high safe dose

Safe-dose range is 115 to 345 mg.
Ordered dose—24 hours: 100 × 3 = 300 mg.
Decision: Give. Within safe-dose range.

2. Estimated wt: 16
   Actual wt:

   Know   **Want to know**

   2.2 lb:1 kg::33:x kg   PROOF: $2.2 \times 15 = 33$
   $2.2x = 33$ $1 \times 33 = 33$
   $x = 15$ kg

   Recommended dose—24 hours:

   Know   **Want to know**

   100:1::x μg:15 kg   PROOF: $100 \times 15 = 1500$
   $x = 1500$ μg—low safe dose $1 \times 1500 = 1500$

   200:1::x μg:15 kg   PROOF: $200 \times 15 = 3000$
   $x = 3000$ μg—high safe dose $1 \times 3000 = 3000$

   Safe-dose range is 1500 μg to 3000 μg.
   Ordered dose—24 hours: 0.5 mg $\times 3 = 1.5$ mg or 1500 μg.
   Decision: Give. Within safe-dose range.

3. Estimated wt: 10 kg
   Actual wt:

   Know   **Want to know**

   2.2 lb:1 kg::20 lb:x kg   PROOF: $2.2 \times 9.1 = 20.0$
   $2.2x = 20$ $1 \times 20 = 20$
   $x = 9.09$ or 9.1 kg

   Recommended dose—24 hours:

   Know   **Want to know**

   2 mg:1 kg::x mg:9.1 kg   PROOF: $2 \times 9.1 = 18.2$
   $x = 2 \times 9.1$ or 18.2 mg—low safe dose $1 \times 18.2 = 18.2$

   4 mg:1 kg::x mg:9.1 kg   PROOF: $4 \times 9.1 = 36.4$
   $x = 2.5 \times 9.1$ or 36.4 mg $1 \times 36.4 = 36.4$

   Safe-dose range is 18.2 to 36.4 mg.
   Ordered dose—24 hours: 50 mg.
   Decision: Hold and clarify promptly. Overdose.

4. Estimated wt: 2.5 kg
   Actual wt:

   Know   **Want to know**

   2.2 lb:1 kg::5 lb:x kg   PROOF: $2.2 \times 2.27 = 4.99$ or 5
   $2.2x = 5$ $1 \times 5 = 5$
   $x = 2.27$ or 2.3 kg

   Recommended dose—24 hours:

Know   Want to know

10 µg:1 kg::x µg:2.3 kg

x = 2.3 × 10 or 23 µg—low safe dose

PROOF: 10 × 2.3 = 23

1 × 24 = 24

Know   Want to know

20 µg:1 kg::x µg:2.3 kg

x = 2.3 × 20 or 46 µg—high safe dose

PROOF: 20 × 2.3 = 46

1 × 46 = 46

Safe dose range is 23 to 46 µg/day.

Ordered dose—24 hours: 0.03 × 4 = 0.12 mg/day or 120 µg/day.

Decision: Hold and clarify promptly. Overdose.

5.   Estimated wt: 42 kg
     Actual wt:

Know   Want to know

2.2 lb:1 kg::85 lb:x kg

2.2x = 85

x = 38.63 or 38.6 kg

PROOF: 2.2 × 38.6 = 84.9 or 85

1 × 85 = 85

Recommended dose—24 hours:

Know   Want to know

10 mg:1 kg::x mg:38.6 kg

x = 38.6 × 10 or 386 mg/day—low safe dose

PROOF: 10 × 38.6 = 38.6

1 × 38.6 = 38.6

Know   Want to know

15 mg:1 kg::x mg:38.6 kg

x = 38.6 × 15 or 579 mg/day—high safe dose

PROOF: 15 × 38.6 = 579

1 × 579 = 579

Safe dose range is 386 to 567 mg/day.

Ordered dose—24 hours: 100 × 4 or 400 mg daily.

Decision: Give. Within safe-dose range.

□ **9C**   (p. 139)

1.   Estimated weight: 19 kg
     lb to kg
     Actual weight:

Know   Want to know

2.2 lb:1 kg::39.6:x kg

2.2x = 39.6

x = 18 lb

PROOF: 2.2 × 18 = 39.6

1 × 39.6 = 39.6

Recommended dose:

Know   Want to know

5:1:: x:18

1x = 5 × 18

x = 90 mg/day

PROOF: 5 × 18 = 90

1 × 90 = 90

Ordered: 30 mg × 3 = 90 mg/day.
Decision: give. 1.2 ml—within safe range.

Have   **Want to have**

125 mg:5 ml::30 mg:x ml   PROOF: 125 × 1.2 = 150
125x = 5 × 30 or 150   5 × 30 = 150
x = 1.2 ml

2. Estimated weight 6 kg
    lb to kg
    Actual weight:

Know   **Want to know**

2.2 lb:1 kg::12.3 lb:x kg   PROOF: 2.2 × 5.6 = 12.3
2.2x = 12.3 × 1 or 5.6 kg   1 × 12.3 = 12.3

Recommended dose:

Know   **Want to know**

100 mg:1 kg::x mg:5.6 kg   PROOF: 100 × 5.6 = 560
1x = 100 × 5.6 = 560 mg—low safe dose   1 × 560 = 560

Know   **Want to know**

200 mg:1 kg::x mg:5.6 kg   PROOF: 200 × 5.6 = 1120
x = 200 × 5.6 or 1120 mg/day—high safe dose   1 × 1320 = 1120

Safe-dose range is 560 to 1120 mg/day.
Ordered: 200 mg × 4 = 800 mg/day.
Decision: give. 8 ml—within safe range.

Have   **Want to have**

125 mg:5 ml::200 mg:x ml   PROOF: 125 × 8 = 1000
125x = 1000   5 × 200 = 1000
x = 8 ml

3. Estimated weight: 31 kg
    lb to kg
    Actual weight:

Know   **Want to know**

2.2 kg:1 lb::62:x kg   PROOF: 2.2 × 28.2 = 62
2.2x = 1 × 62   1 × 62 = 62
x = 28.2

Recommended dose:

Know   **Want to know**

6 mg:1 kg::x mg:28.2 kg   PROOF: 6 × 28.2 = 169.2
1x = 6 × 28.2 or 169.2 mg—low safe dose   1 × 169.2 = 169.2

Know   **Want to know**

12 mg:1 kg::x mg:28.2 kg   PROOF: 12 × 28.2 = 338.4

1x = 12 × 28.2 or 338.4 mg—high safe dose   1 × 338.4 = 338.4

Safe dose range is 169.2 to 338.4 mg daily.
Ordered dose: 300 mg × 3 = 900 mg/day.
Decision: hold and clarify promptly. Overdose.

4.   Estimated weight: 25 kg
     lb to kg
     Actual weight:

    Know   **Want to know**

    2.2 lb:1 kg::50 lb:x kg   PROOF: 2.2 × 22.7 = 50

    2.2x = 1 × 50   1 × 50 = 50

    x = 22.7 kg

    Recommended dose:

    Know   **Want to know**

    240 mg:1 kg::x mg:22.7 kg   PROOF: 240 × 22.7 = 5448

    1x = 240 × 22.7 or 5448 mg or 5.4 g—low safe dose   1 × 5448 = 5448

    Know   **Want to know**

    360 mg:1 kg::x mg:22.7 kg   PROOF: 360 × 22.7 = 8172

    1x = 360 × 22.7 or 8172 mg or 8.2 g—High safe dose   1 × 8172 = 8172

    Safe dose range is 5448 mg or 5.4 g to 8172 mg or 8.2 g.
    Ordered dose: 2000 mg × 3 or 6000 mg/day.
    Decision: give 4 tablets. Within safe range.

    Have   **Want to have**

    0.5 g:1 tablet::2 g:x tablet   PROOF: 0.5 × 4 = 2

    0.5x = 2   1 × 2 = 2

    x = 4 tablets

5.   Weight in m^2 for 30-lb child is 0.6 m^2 on BSA nomogram.
     lb to kg
     Recommended dose:

    Know   **Want to know**

    40:1 m^2::x mg:0.6 m^2 PROOF: 40 × 0.6 = 24

    x = 24 mg   1 × 24 = 24

    Ordered dose: 20 mg.
    Decision: Give 2 tablets. Safe dose. Slightly below recommended dose.

1. Estimated wt: 2.5 kg
   oz to lb:

   Know   Want to know
   16 oz:1 lb::10 oz:x lb   PROOF*: 16 × .6 = 9.6 or 10
   16x = 10   1 × 10 = 10
   x = 0.62 or 0.6 lb

   lb to kg:
   2.2 lb:1 kg::5.6 lb:x kg   PROOF*: 2.2 × 2.54 = 5.58 or 5.6
   2.2x = 1 × 5.6   1 × 5.6 = 5.6

   Actual wt:
   x = 2.54 or 2.5 kg

   Recommended dose:
   50 mg:1 kg::x mg:2.5 kg   PROOF: 50 × 2.5 = 125
   x = 50 × 2.5 or 125 mg daily in divided doses   1 × 125 = 125

   Ordered: 75 mg × 3 = 225 mg daily.
   Decision: Hold and clarify. Overdose.

2. Estimated wt: 4 kg
   oz to lb:
   16 oz:1 lb::2 oz:x lb   PROOF*: 16 × .12 = 1.9 or 2
   16x = 2   1 × 2 = 2
   x = .12 or .1 lb

   lb to kg:
   2.2 lb:1 kg::9.1 lb:x kg   PROOF*: 2.2 × 4.13 = 9.08 or 9.1
   2.2x = 1 × 9.1   1 × 9.1 = 9.1

   Actual wt:
   x = 4.13 or 4.1 kg

   Recommended dose:
   20 mg:1kg::x mg:4.1 kg   PROOF*: 20 × 4.1 = 82
   x = 20 × 4.1 or 82 mg bid or 164 daily   1 × 82 = 82

   Ordered:
   40 mg bid or 80 mg daily

   Decision:
   Give 0.13 ml and clarify. Low dose.

---

*Rounding will cause proofs to be inexact.

Have   Want to have

300 mg:1 ml::40 mg:x ml

$300x = 1 \times 40$

$x = 0.133$ ml or 0.13 ml

PROOF: $300 \times 0.133 = 39.9$

$1 \times 40 = 40$

3. Estimated wt: 9 kg
    Actual wt:

Know   Want to know

2.2 lb:1 kg::18 lb:x kg

$2.2x = 18$

$x = 8.18$ or 8.2 kg

PROOF: $2.2 \times 8.2 = 18$

$1 \times 18 = 18$

Recommended dose:

Know   Want to know

2 mg:1 kg:x mg:8.2 kg

$x = 2 \times 8.2$ or 16.4 mg—low safe dose

PROOF: $2 \times 8.2 = 16.4$

$1 \times 16.4 = 16.4$

2.5 mg:1 kg::x mg:8.2 kg

$x = 2.5 \times 8.2$ or 20.5 mg—high safe dose

PROOF: $2.5 \times 8.2 = 20.5$

$1 \times 20.5 = 20.5$

Safe-dose range: 16.4 to 20.5 mg q8h (tid).
Ordered: 20 mg tid.

Decision:
Give 2 ml injectable.

Have   Want to have

10 mg:1 ml::20 mg:x ml

$10x = 20$

$x = 2$ ml

PROOF: $10 \times 2 = 20$

$1 \times 20 = 20$

4. Estimated wt: 10 kg
    Actual wt:

Know   Want to know

2.2 lb:1 kg::20.5 lb:x kg

$2.2x = 1 \times 20.5$

$x = 9.31$ or 9.3 kg

PROOF: $2.2 \times 9.31 = 20.48$

$1 \times 20.5 = 20.5$

Recommended dose:

Know   Want to know

1 mg:1 kg:x mg:9.3 kg

$x = 9.3$ mg—low safe dose

2.2 mg:1 kg:x mg:9.3 kg

$x = 9.3 \times 2.2$ or 20.5 mg—high safe dose

PROOF: $2.1 \times 9.3 = 20.46$ or 20.5

$1 \times 10.5 = 20.5$

Safe-dose range: 9.3 mg to 20.5 mg.
Ordered dose: 15 mg

Decision:
Safe. Give 0.6 ml.

Have   Want to have

25 mg:1 ml::15 mg:x ml   PROOF: 25 × 0.6 = 15
25x = 15   1 × 15 = 15
x = 0.6 ml

5. Estimated wt: 20 kg
    Actual weight:

Know   Want to know

2.2 lb:1 kg::40 lb:x kg   PROOF: 2.2 × 18.2 = 40
2.2x = 20   1 × 40 = 40
x = 18.18 or 18.2 kg

Recommended dose:

Know   Want to know

2.2 mg:1 kg::x mg:18.2 kg   PROOF: 2.2 × 18.2 = 40.0
x = 2.2 × 18.2 or 40.0 mg—low safe dose   1 × 40 = 40

Know   Want to know

4.4 mg:1 kg::x mg:18.2 kg   PROOF: 4.4 × 18.2 = 80
x = 4.4 × 18.2 or 80 mg—high safe dose   1 × 80 = 80

Safe-dose range: 40 to 80 mg/day.
Ordered: 20 mg bid or 40 mg/day.
Decision:
Safe. Give 0.4 ml.

Have   Want to have

50 mg:1 ml::20 mg:x ml   PROOF: 50 × 0.4 = 20
50x = 20   1 × 20 = 20
x = 0.4 ml

□ **9E**   (p. 143)

1. Estimated wt: 3.5 kg
    Actual wt:

Know   Want to know

16 oz:1 lb::2 oz:x lb   PROOF*: 16 × .12 = 1.9 or 2
16 x = 2   1 × 2 = 2
x = .12 lb

Know   Want to know

2.2 lb:1 kg::7.1:x kg

2.2x = 1 × 7.1

x = 3.2 kg

Recommended dose:

Know   Want to know

3 mg:1 kg::x mg:3.2 kg   PROOF: 3 × 3.2 = 9.6

1x = 3 × 3.2 or 9.6 mg—low safe dose   1 × 9.6 = 9.6

Know   Want to know

6 mg:1 kg::x mg:3.2 kg   PROOF: 6 × 3.2 = 19.2

1x = 6 × 3.2 or 19.2 mg—high safe dose   1 × 19.2 = 19.2

Safe-dose range: 9.6 to 19.2 mg q24h.

Ordered dose: 10 mg q6h or 40 mg q24h.

Decision: Hold and clarify promptly. Overdose.

2.   Estimated wt.: 24 kg

Actual wt:

Know   Want to know

2.2 lb:1 kg::48 lb:x kg   PROOF: 2.2 × 21.8 = 47.9 or 48

2.2x = 48   1 × 48 = 48

x = 21.8 kg

Recommended dose: 1 to 6 mg/kg

Know   Want to know

1 mg:1 kg::x mg:21.8 kg   PROOF: 1 × 21.8 = 21.8

1x = 21.8 mg—low safe dose   1 × 21.8 = 21.8

Know   Want to know

6 mg:1 kg::x mg:21.8 kg   PROOF: 6 × 21.8 = 130.8

6x = 21.8   1 × 21.8 = 130.8

x = 130.8 mg—high safe dose

Safe-dose range: 21.8 to 130.8 mg.

Ordered dose: 150 mg.

Decision:

Hold and clarify promptly—overdose.

---

*Proofs will be exact if carried to second or third decimal place.

3. Estimated wt: 17 kg
    Actual wt:

    Know   **Want to know**
    2.2 lb:1 kg::35 lb:x kg
    $2.2x = 35$
    $x = 15.9$ kg
    Recommended dose:

    Know   **Want to know**
    15 μg:1 kg::x μg:15.9 kg
    $x = 15 \times 15.9$ or 238.5 μg/day

    Ordered dose: 0.20 mg

    Know   **Want to know**
    1000 μg:1 mg::238.5 μg:x mg   PROOF: $1000 \times .238 = 238$
    $1000x = 238.5$ $1 \times 238.5 = 238.5$
    $x = .238$ mg or 0.2 mg

    Decision:
    Give 0.4 ml. Safe dose.

    Have   **Want to have**
    0.5 mg:1 ml::0.2 mg:x ml   PROOF: $0.5 \times 0.4 = 0.2$
    $0.5x = 0.2$ $1 \times 0.2 = 0.2$
    $x = 0.4$ ml

4. Estimated wt: 13 kg
    Actual wt:

    Know   **Want to know**
    2.2 lb:1 kg::26 lb:x kg   PROOF: $2.2 \times 11.8 = 26$
    $2.2x = 26$ $1 \times 26 = 26$
    $x = 11.8$ kg

    Recommended dose:

    Know   **Want to know**
    0.03 mg:1 kg::x mg:11.8 kg   PROOF: $0.03 \times 11.8 = 0.35$
    $x = 11.8 \times 0.03$ $1 \times 0.35 = 0.35$
    $x = 0.35$ mg—low safe dose

    Know   **Want to know**
    0.05 mg:1 kg::x mg:11.8 kg   PROOF: $0.05 \times 11.8 = 0.59$
    $x = 11.8 \times 0.05$ $1 \times 0.59 = 0.59$
    $x = 0.59$ mg—high safe dose

Safe dose range: 0.35 to 0.59 mg.
Ordered dose: 0.7 mg.
Decision: Hold and clarify promptly. Overdose.

5. Estimated wt: 17 kg
    Actual wt:

    Know   **Want to know**
    2.2 lb:1 kg::35 lb:x kg   PROOF: 2.2 × 15.9 = 35.9 or 35
    2.2x = 35   1 × 15.9 = 35
    x = 15.9 kg

    Recommended dose:

    Know   **Want to know**
    40 mg:1 kg::x mg:15.9 kg   PROOF: 40 × 15.9 = 636
    x = 40 × 15.9 or 636 mg—low safe dose   1 × 636 = 636

    Know   **Want to know**
    80 mg:1 kg::x mg:15.9 kg   PROOF: 80 × 15.9 = 1272
    x = 80 × 15.9 or 1272 mg—high safe dose   1 × 1272 = 1272

    Safe dose range: 636 to 1272 mg.
    Ordered dose: 0.25 g q6h or 250 mg q6h or 1000 mg in 24 hours.
    Decision:
    Give 2.5 ml. Within safe-dose range.

    Have   **Want to have**
    1 g:10 ml::0.25 g:x ml   PROOF: 1 × 2.5 = 2.5
    x = 2.5 ml   10 × 0.25 = 2.5

CHAPTER 9

Children's Dosages Test   (p. 146)

1. Safe range is 204.5 to 409 mg daily.
    Safe order; withdraw 4 ml.
2. Safe dose range is 736 to 1472 mg. Withdraw 1 ml from vial for 250 mg/dose.
3. Safe dosage is 22.8 mg. Order is safe at 20 mg. Give 2 ml po stat.
4. Safe dose range is 27.3 to 163.8 mg.
    Ordered dose is safe at 30 mg. Give 1.5 ml.
5. Safe dose range is 0.6 to 1 mg.
    Ordered dose is safe at 0.8 mg. Give 1.6 ml.
6. Give 180 mg or 54.5 ml.*

*Refer to BSA mg/m^2 method, p. 132.

7. 500 mg. Give 10 ml or 2 tsp.
8. Measure 3.75 ml. Measure one full dropper with 2.5 ml and then measure to 1.25 ml calibration on the dropper again to complete the dose.
9. Each teaspoon will contain 250 mg.
10. 54 mg

CHAPTER 10

Advanced intravenous calculations

☐ **10A**   (p. 154)

1. a. 1500 μg/hr or 1.5 mg/hr
   b. 9600 μg/hr or 9.6 mg/hr
   c. 9900 μg or 9.9 mg/hr
   d. 12,000 μg/hr or 12 mg/hr
   e. 72,000 μg/hr or 72 mg/hr

2. a. 1:4
   b. 1:1
   c. 1:10
   d. 1:2
   e. 1:2

3. a. $x = 40$ ml/hr (1:4::10:40)
   b. $x = 30$ ml/hr (1:1::30:30)
   c. $x = 50$ ml/hr (1:10::5:50)
   d. $x = 6$ ml/hr (1:2::3:6)
   e. $x = 5$ ml/hr (2:1::10:5)

4. a. 20 mg
   b. 12 mg
   c. 9 mg
   d. 4 mg
   e. 36 mg

5. a. 16 ml/hr (1:4::4:16)
   b. 9 ml/hr (1:1::9:9)
   c. 10 ml/hr (2:1::20:10)
   d. 30 ml/hr (1:2::1:2)
   e. 5 ml/hr (8:5::8:5)

☐ **10B**   (p. 156)

1. *Step 1—safe range*

   Know   Want to know

   2 μg:1 kg::x μg:50 kg   PROOF: 2 × 50 = 100
   $x = 2 × 50$ or 100 μg/min—low safe dose   1 × 100 = 100

   5 μg:1 kg::x μg:50 kg   PROOF: 5 × 50 = 250
   $x = 5 × 50$ or 250 μg/min—high safe dose   1 × 250 = 250

   Step 2—comparison of order with range in literature
   Order of 75 μg/min is below safe range. Clarify order.

   Step 3—hourly drug order and hourly flow rate

   a. 75 μg/min × 60 = 4500 μg/hr or 4.5 mg/hr

b. Total drug:total volume::hourly drug:hourly volume

      250 mg: 250 ml   PROOF: $1 \times 4.5 = 4.5$

          1:           1::   4.5 mg:x ml/hr $1 \times 4.5 = 4.5$

$x = 1 \times 4.5 = 4.5$ or 5 ml/hr

2. *Step 1—hourly drug order in μg and mg*
100 μg $\times$ 60 = 6000 μg/hr or 6 mg/hr

Step 2—hourly flow rate
Total drug:total volume::hourly drug:hourly volume

      250 mg: 250 ml   PROOF: $1 \times 6 = 6$

          1:        1 ml::   6 mg:x ml/hr $1 \times 6 = 6$

$x = 6$ ml hr

Step 3
Flow rate is incorrect at 5 ml/hr. Change to 6 ml/hr.

3. *Step 1—mg/hr*
4 mg $\times$ 60 = 240 mg/hr*

Step 2—flow rate
Total drug:total volume::hourly drug:hourly volume

    1000 mg: 500 ml::   240 mg:x ml   PROOF: $2 \times 120 = 240$

         2:         1::   240 mg:x $1 \times 240 = 240$

$2x = 240$
$x = 120$ ml/hr

4. *Step 1—safe-dose range*
150 lb = 68.2 kg

2.5 μg:1 kg::xμg:68.2 kg   PROOF: $2.5 \times 68.2 = 170.5$
$x = 2.5 \times 68.2$ $1 \times 170.5 = 170.5$
$x = 170.5$ μg—low safe dose/min

10 μg:1 kg::x μg:68.2 kg   PROOF: $10 \times 68.2 = 682$
$x = 682$ μg maximum safe dose/min $1 \times 682 = 682$
safe-dose range is 170.5 to 682 μg/min

Step 2
100 μg/min is low for this patient.
Call and clarify the order.

5. *Step 1—μg/hr and mg/hr*
500 μg/min $\times$ 60 = 30,000 μg/hr or 30 mg/hr*

---

*Use of a calculator simplifies conversions.

Step 2—ml/hr
Total drug:total volume::hourly drug:hourly volume
    500 mg: 500 ml
      1 mg: 1 ml::   30 mg:x ml/hr
x = 30 ml/hr. The flowrate is correct.

Step 3—μg/hr and mg/hr
150 μg/min × 60 = 9000 μg/hr or 9 mg/hr

Step 4—ml/hr
Total drug:total volume::hourly drug:hourly volume
    500 mg: 500 ml
      1 mg: 1 ml::   9 mg:x ml
x = 9 ml an hour. Reduce flow from 30 to 9 ml/hr.

□ **10C**   (p. 157)

1. 2 mg/min = 120 mg/hr

    Total drug:total volume::hourly drug:hourly volume
            1 g: 500 ml   PROOF: 2 × 60 = 60
       1000 mg: 500 ml   1 × 60 = 60
          2 mg: 1 ml::   120 mg:x ml/hr
    $2x$ = 120
    x = 60 ml/hour

2. *Step 1—μg/min to μg/hr*
    (Ratio or use calculator)

    5 μg:1 min::x μg:60 min   PROOF: 1 × 1.5 = 1.5
    x = 5 × 60 or 300 μg/hour   5 × 0.3 = 1.5

    Step 2—ml/hr
    Total drug:total volume::hourly drug:hourly volume
        50 mg: 250 ml   PROOF: 1 × 3 = 3
         5 mg: 25 ml   5 × 0.6 = 3
         1 mg: 5 ml::300 μg or 0.3 mg:x ml
    x = 5 × 0.3 mg
    x = 1.5 or 2 ml/hr

3. *Step 1—safe range*

    Know   **Want to know**
    2 μg:1 kg::x μg:50 kg   PROOF: 2 × 50 = 100
    x = 2 × 50 or 100 μg/min—low safe dose   1 × 100 = 100

    Know   **Want to know**
    5 μg:1 kg::x μg:50 kg   PROOF: 5 × 50 = 250
    x = 5 × 50 or 250 μg/min—high safe dose   1 × 250 = 250

Safe-dose range is 100 to 250 µg/min.
Order to 150 µg/min is within safe range.

Step 2—mg/hr ordered
Use calculator and then move decimal three places to left to change µg to mg.
150 µg × 60 or 9000 µg/hr = 9 mg/hr

Step 3—ml/hr
Total drug:total volume::hourly drug:hourly volume
    250 mg: 250 ml::   in mg
      1 mg: 1 ml::   9 mg:x ml
x = 9 ml/hr

4. *Step 1—drug/min ordered*

  Know   **Want to know**
  5 µg:1 kg::x µg:80 kg
  x = 5 × 80 or 400 µg/min

  Step 2—Hourly drug in mg ordered
  400 × 60 min = 24,000 µg/hr or 24 mg/hour

  Step 3—ml/hour ordered
  Total drug:total volume::hourly drug:hourly volume   PROOF: 1 × 48 = 48
     250 mg: 500 ml   2 × 24 = 48
       1 mg: 2 ml::   24 mg:x ml/hr
  x = 2 × 24 or 48 ml/hr

  Flow rate at 24 ml/hr is incorrect. Reset to 48 ml/hr.

5. *Step 1—Wt in kg*
  154 lb = 70 kg

  Step 2—Safe-dose range

  Know   **Want to know**
  0.5 µg:1 kg::x µg:70 kg
  x = 35 µg—low safe dose per minute

  Know   **Want to know**
  10 µg:1 kg::x µg:70 kg
  x = 700 µg—high safe dose per minute

  Safe-dose range is 35 to 700 µg/min.
  Comparison of order with safe dose range.

  Order is 0.25 mg/min or 250 µg/min.
  Order is within safe-dose range.

  Step 3—mg and ml/hr ordered
  0.25 mg/min = 15 mg/hr (0.25 × 60)

Total drug:total volume::hourly drug:hourly volume

			PROOF: $1 \times 75 = 75$
50 mg:	250 ml		
1 mg:	5 ml::	15 mg:x ml/hr	$5 \times 15 = 75$

$x = 75$ ml/hr

☐ **10D**   (p. 158)

1. *Step 1—reduced ratio*
   Total drug:total volume
   40 g:1000 ml
   4:100
   1:25—lowest reduced ratio

   Step 2—ml/hr

   Know   **Want to know**
   Total drug:total volume::hourly drug:hourly volume

			PROOF: $40 \times 50 = 2000$
40 g:	1000 ml::	2 g:x ml/hr	
1:	25 ml::	2 g:x ml/hr	$1000 \times 2 = 2000$

   $x = 25 \times 2$
   $x = 50$ ml hour

2. *Step 1—lowest reduced ratio*

   Know
   10 u:1000
   1:100—reduced ratio

   Step 2—recommended dose

   Know   **Want to know**
   20 mU:1 min::x mu:60 min*
   $x = 20 \times 60$ PROOF: $20 \times 60 = 1200$
   $x = 1200$ mU/hour or 1.2 u/hour†—safe high dose $1 \times 1200 = 1200$

Know   **Want to know**
1000 mu:1 u::1200 mU:x u   PROOF: $1000 \times 1.2 = 1200$
$1000x = 1200$ or 1.2 u an hour $1 \times 1200 = 1200$

---

*To change mU to u, move decimal three places to left.
†Multiply minute dose by 60 with a calculator.

Step 3—hourly drug ordered

Know   **Want to know**

Total drug:total volume::hourly drug:hourly volume

        10 u: 1000 ml:: x u:100 ml

Reduced ratio   1:   100:: x u:100 ml

$x = 1$ u/hr

PROOF: $1 \times 100 = 100$

$1 \times 100 = 100$

Decision: 1 u/hr is safe dose. Does not exceed recommended dose.

3. *Step 1—mU/hr*

    Know   **Want to know**

    2 mU:1 min::x mU:60 min   PROOF: $2 \times 60 = 120$

    $x = 2$ (60) or 120 mU/hr $1 \times 120 = 120$

    Step 2—mU/hr to U/hr

    Know   **Want to know**

    1000 mU:1 U::120 mU:x U

    $1000x = 120$ PROOF: $1000 \times 0.12 = 120$

    $x = 120/1000$ or 0.12 U/hr (decimal moved three to left) $1 \times 120 = 120$

Step 3—hourly volume (ml/hr)

Total drug:total volume::hour drug:hourly volume

20 U:1000::0.12 U:x ml/hr   PROOF: $20 \times 6 = 120$

Reduced ratio   1:50 $1000 \times .12 = 120$

$x = 0.12(50)$

$x = 6$ ml/hr will be infused

4. *Step 1—lowest reduced ratio*

    Total drug:total volume

    20 g:500 ml

    2:50

    1:25—lowest reduced ratio

    Step 2—g/hr (hourly drug) to be infused

    Know   **Want to know**

    Total drug:total volume::hourly drug:hourly volume

    20:500

    1 g:25 ml::x g:25 ml

    $25x = 25$ PROOF: $1 \times 25 = 25$

    $25x = 25 = 1$ g/hr $1 \times 25 = 25$

Step 3—time for 4 g to be infused

Know   **Want to know**

1 g:1 hour::4 g:x hours

$x = 4$

$x = 4$ hours for 4 g to be infused

PROOF: 1 × 4 = 4
1 × 4 = 4

5. *Step 1—lowest reduced ratio*
    40 g:250 ml
    4:25—lowest reduced ratio

    Step 2—ml/hr ordered

    Know   **Want to know**

    Total drug:total volume::hourly drug:hourly volume
    40 g::250 ml
    4:25 ml::2 g:x ml/hour
    $4x = 50$
    $x = 12.5$ or 13 ml/hour ordered (must use nearest whole number)

PROOF: 4 × 12.5 = 50
25 × 2 = 50

    Step 3
    Incorrect flow rate at 25 ml/hr. Report promptly and readjust to 13 ml/hr.

☐ **10E**   (p. 160)

1. *Step 1—safe-dose range*

    Know   **Want to know**

    0.1 mg:1 kg::x µg:60 kg
    $0.1x = 60$
    $x = 6$ mg/hr—low safe dose

PROOF: 0.1 × 60 = 6
1 × 60 = 6

    0.5 mg:1 kg:x mg:60 kg
    $x = 60 × 0.5$
    $x = 30$ mg/hr—high safe dose

PROOF: 0.5 × 60 = 30
1 × 30 = 30

    Safe-dose range for 60 kg patient is 6 to 30 mg/hr.

    Step 2—lowest reduced ratio

    Know

    Total drug:total volume
    250 mg:1000 ml
    25:100
    1:4—lowest reduced ratio

Step 3—mg/hr
Total drug*:total volume::hourly drug:hourly volume
250 mg:1000 ml
1:4 ::x mg:50
$4x = 50$ PROOF: $1 \times 50 = 50$
$x = 12.5$ mg/hr $4 \times 12.5 = 50$

Decision: Administer—12.5 is within safe range.

2. *Step 1—safe-dose range for 80 kg patient*

   Know   **Want to know**
   0.5 mg:1 kg::x mg:80 kg   PROOF: $0.5 \times 80 = 40$
   $x = 80 \times 0.5$ or 40 mg/hr—low safe dose $1 \times 40 = 40$

   Know   **Want to know**
   0.7 mg:1 kg::x mg:80 kg   PROOF: $0.7 \times 80 = 56$
   $x = 0.7 \times 80$ or 56 mg/hr—high safe dose $1 \times 56 = 56$

   Safe-dose range for 80 kg patient is 40 to 56 mg/hr.

   Step 2
   45 mg/hr is within safe range for this patient.

   Step 3—reduced ratio of total drug to total volume

   Know
   500 mg:1000
   50:100
   5:10
   1:2—lowest reduced ratio

   Step 4—ml/hr or hourly volume
   Total drug:total volume::hourly drug:hourly volume
   500 mg:1000 ml
   1:2 ml::45 mg:x ml/hr   PROOF: $1 \times 90 = 90$
   $x = 90$ ml/hr. Infuse. $45 \times 2 = 90$

3. *Step 1—safe dose range*

   Know   **Want to know**
   0.1 mg:1 kg::x mg:70 kg   PROOF: $0.1 \times 70 = 7$
   $x = 7$ mg/hr—low safe dose $1 \times 7 = 7$

   0.5 mg:1 kg::x mg:70 kg   PROOF: $0.5 \times 70 = 35$
   $x = 35$ mg/hr—high safe dose $1 \times 35 = 35$

---

*Labeling helps prevent errors.

Step 2—reduced ratio of total drug to total volume
250 mg:500 ml
1:2 ml—lowest reduced ratio

Step 3—mg/hr
Total drug:total volume::hourly drug:hourly volume
250 mg:500 ml
1 mg:2 ml::x mg:50 ml
$2x = 50$ PROOF: $1 \times 50 = 50$
$x = 25$ mg/hr $2 \times 25 = 50$

Step 4
25 mg/hr is within safe range for a 70 kg patient

4. *Step 1—maximum safe dose*

    Know   Want to know
    0.5 mg:1 kg::x mg:50 kg
    $x = 0.5 \times 50$ or 25 mg/hr—maximum safe maintenance dose

    Step 2
    20 mg/hr is safe order for this patient.

    Step 3—reduced ratio of total drug to total volume

            Know
    250 mg:500 ml
       1 mg:2 ml–lowest reduced ratio

    Step 4—ml/hour
    Total drug:total volume::hourly drug:hourly volume
    250 mg:500 ml
    1 mg:2 ml::20 mg:x ml/hr
    $x = 2 \times 20$ or 40 ml/hr (Were you able to do this without calculation?)

5. *Step 1—safe range*

    Know   Want to know
    2.2 lb:1 kg::154 lb:x kg
    $2.2x = 154$
    $x = 70$ kg (patient weight)

    Know   Want to know
    0.1 mg:1 kg::x mg:70 kg
    $x = 7$ mg/hr—low safe dose

    0.5 mg:1 kg::x mg:70 kg
    $x = 35$ mg/hr—maximum safe dose

    Decision: 15 mg/hr ordered is safe dose.

5. *Step 2 ml/hr ordered*

   Know   **Want to know**

   Total drug:total volume::hourly drug:hourly volume
   500 mg:1000 ml
   1:2 ::15 mg:x ml/hr
   $x = 15 \times 2$ or 30 ml/hr ordered

   Step 3
   Flow rate of 50 ml/hour is too high. Set at 30 ml/hr and report.

☐ **10F**   (p. 164)

1. Total volume:total minutes::x volume:1 min
   20 ml:10 min::x ml:1 min   PROOF: $20 \times 1 = 20$
   $10x = 20$ $10 \times 2 = 20$
   $x = 2$ ml/min or 1 ml/30 sec

2. *Step 1—total volume*

   Know   **Want to know**

   250 μg:1 ml::1000 μg (1 mg):x ml   PROOF: $250 \times 4 = 1000$
   $250x = 1000$ $1 \times 1000 = 1000$
   $x = 4$ ml

   Step 2—volume/minute
   Total volume:total minutes::x volume:1 min
   4 ml:10 min::x volume:1 min
   $10x = 4$
   $x = 0.4$ ml q minute or 60 seconds   PROOF: $4 \times 1 = 4$
       0.1 m q 15 seconds $10 \times 0.4 = 4$

3. *Step 1—total volume to be injected*

   Know   **Want to know**

   100 mg:1 ml::900 mg:x ml
   $100x = 900$
   $x = 9$ ml

   Step 2—total minutes

   Know   **Want to know**

   50 mg:1 minute::900 mg:x minutes   PROOF: $50 \times 18 = 900$
   $50x = 900$ $1 \times 900 = 900$
   $x = 18$ minutes total time

Step 3—minute volume

Total volume:total minutes::minute volume:1 minute

(ml/min)

9 ml:18 min   PROOF: $1 \times 1 = 1$
1 ml:2 min:x ml:1 min $2 \times 0.5 = 1$
$2x = 1$
$x = 0.5$ ml/min or 60 seconds
    0.25 ml/½ min or 30 seconds

4. Total volume:total minutes::minute volume:1 minute
   2 ml:10 min
   1 ml:5 min::x ml:1 min
   $5x = 1$ PROOF: $1 \times 1 = 1$
   $x = 0.2$ ml/min $5 \times 0.2 = 1$

5. Total volume:total minutes::minute volume:1 minute
   5 ml:5 min   PROOF: $1 \times 1 = 1$
   1 :1::x ml:1 min $1 \times 1 = 1$
   $x = 1$ ml/min

CHAPTER 11

Solutions

□ **11A**   (p. 167)

1. **Have   Want**

   0.9 g:100 ml::x g NaC1:500 ml water   PROOF: $0.9 \times 500 = 450$
   $100x = 450$ $100 \times 4.5 = 450$
   $x = 4.5$ g salt added to 500 ml water

   REMEMBER: 1 tsp = 4 to 5 ml or g

2. **Have   Want**

   0.9:100::x g NaCl:200   PROOF: $0.9 \times 200 = 180$
   $100x = 180$ $100 \times 1.8 = 180$
   $x = 1.8$ g salt added to 200 ml water

3. **Have   Want**

   5 ml:100 ml::x ml acetic acid:300 ml water   PROOF: $100 \times 15 = 1500$
   $100x = 1500$ $5 \times 300 = 1500$
   $x = 15$ ml acetic acid

Pour 15 ml of 5% acetic acid into a container. Then add water to the 300 ml mark.

300 ml desired
-15 ml acetic acid
285 ml water

4. **Have**   **Want**

10 ml:100 ml::x ml acetic acid:250 ml   PROOF: $10 \times 250 = 2500$
$100x = 2500$ $100 \times 25 = 2500$
$x = 25$ ml acetic acid

Pour 25 ml full-strength acetic acid into container. Then add water to the 250 ml mark.

250 ml desired
-25 ml acetic acid
225 ml water

5. **Have**   **Want**

0.9 g:100 ml::x g salt:150 ml   PROOF: $100 \times 1.35 = 135$
$100x = 135$ $0.9 \times 150 = 135$
$x = 1.35 = 1$ ml or g salt

Add 1 g of salt to 150 ml of water. Because it is difficult to measure 1 g or ml of salt, just make up a normal saline solution of 500 ml water (1 pt) and add 1 tsp (4 to 5 ml) of salt. Discard any unused portion.

6. **Have**   **Want**

10 ml:100 ml::x ml acetic acid:200 ml water   PROOF: $100 \times 20 = 2000$
$100x = 2000$ $10 \times 200 = 2000$
$x = 20$ ml acetic acid

Add 20 ml of 10% acetic acid to the container; add water to make 200 ml.

200 ml desired
-20 ml acetic acid
180 ml water

7. **Have**   **Want**

0.9 g:100 ml::x g NaC1:1000 ml water   PROOF: $100 \times 9 = 900$
$100x = 900$ $0.9 \times 1000 = 900$
$x = 9$ g NaC1 or 2 tsp

Always prepare a 1000-ml solution for an enema.

8. **Have**   **Want**

0.9 g:100 ml::x g NaC1:500 ml water   PROOF: $100 \times 4.5 = 450$

$100x = 450$ $0.9 \times 500 = 450$

$x = 4.5$ g salt = 1 tsp.

You should have this problem memorized by now. REMEMBER: 1 tsp in 1 pint of water gives 500 ml of normal saline solution.

9. **Have**   **Want**

$1\frac{1}{2}$ ml:100 ml::x ml vinegar:1000 ml   PROOF: $100 \times 15 = 1500$

                                                 $1\frac{1}{2} \times 1000 = 1500$

$100x = \dfrac{3}{2} \times 1000 = 1500$

$100x = 1500$

$x = 15$ ml vinegar

Add 15 ml or 3 tsp of vinegar to the 1 L container. Add 985 ml water to make up 1000 ml of solution.

10. **Have**   **Want**

40 ml bet.:100 ml sol::x ml betadine:500 ml normal saline

$100\ x = 40 \times 500 = 20,000$

$1\not0\not0x = 20,0\not0\not0$ PROOF: $100 \times 200 = 20,000$

$x = 200$ ml betadine $40 \times 500 = 20,000$

        500 ml desired

       $\underline{-200\ \text{ml}}$ full-strength betadine

add   300 ml normal saline

CHAPTER 11

Solutions Test   (p. 169)

---

1. *Pour:*   8 ml Lysol

    Add: $\underline{3992\ \text{ml}}$ water

               4000 ml of a 1:500 solution of Lysol

2. *Pour:*   125 ml betadine needed

    Add: $\underline{125\ \text{ml}}$ 0.45% normal saline

              250 ml

This means dissolve gr 30 (or six 5-gr tablets) in 1000 ml of a 1:500 solution.

3. *Pour:*   1.3 ml $KMnO_4$

    Add: $\underline{998.7\ \text{ml}}$

              1000 ml = 1:750 solution

4. Each tablet of $KMnO_4$ contains 1 gr. Dissolve 10½ tablets of $KMnO_4$ (1 gr each) in 500 ml of water to make 500 ml of 1:750 solution.

5. *Pour:*   90 ml peroxide

   Add: <u>210 ml</u> solution
                  300 ml use 0.9% saline

Comprehensive examination   (p. 170)

1.	2 ml dose and 6 ml per day	16.	1.6 ml/hr
2.	6 ml*	17.	Yes. Safe order. Wt 15 kg.
3.	2 tab	18.	0.25 ml
4.	0.4 ml	19.	1.3 ml
5.	2 ml	20.	30 ml
6.	63 ml/hr	21.	25 gtts/min
7.	16 gtt/min	22.	1 suppository
8.	125 ml/hr	23.	100 ml
9.	17 gtt/min	24.	15 ml or 3 tsp
10.	1 ml	25.	2 tab
11.	1.3 ml	26.	121 lb
12.	1.5 ml	27.	Safe order. Give 4 ml.
13.	0.7 ml	28.	70 to 140 mg; safe. Give 1 ml.
14.	2 tab	29.	40 gtt/min
15.	0.5 ml	30.	25 ml/hr

*Divide dose and administer in 2 sites.

INDEX